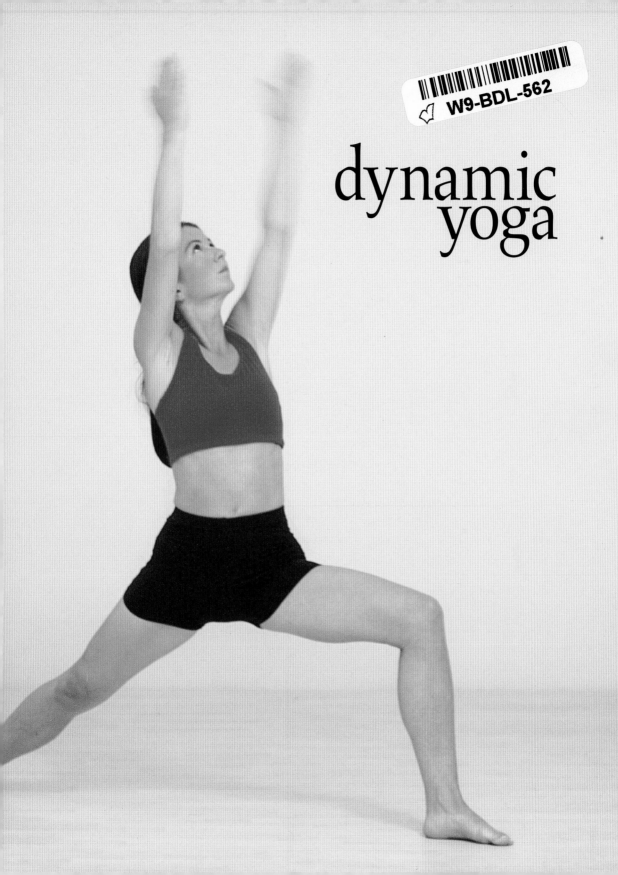

dynamic
yoga

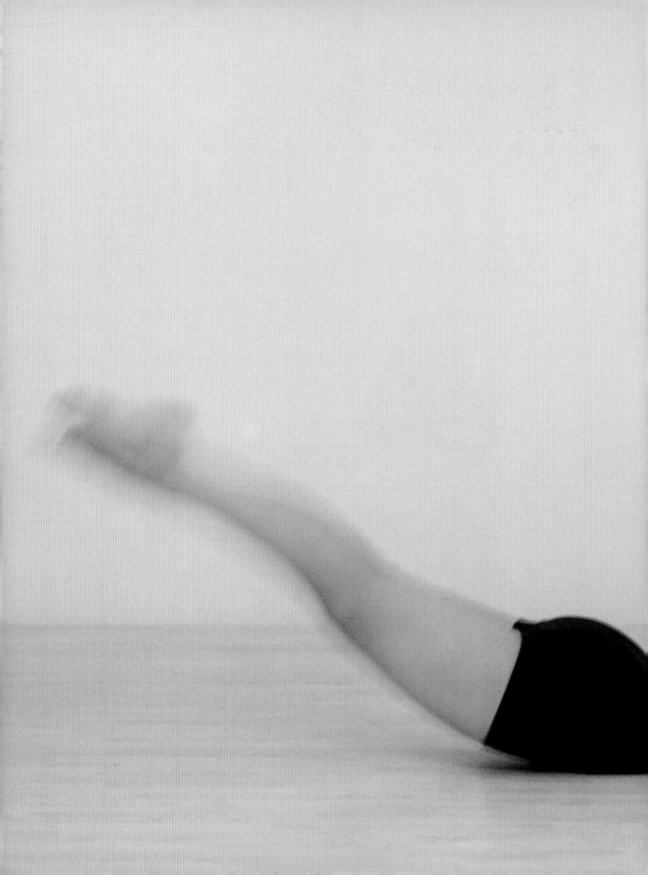

KIA MEAUX
dynamic
yoga

PHOTOGRAPHY BY
RUSSELL SADUR

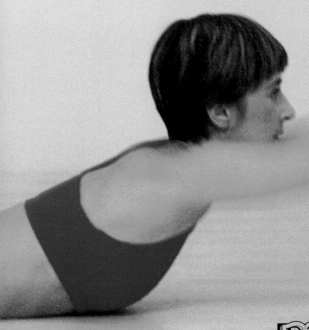

DK

A Dorling Kindersley Book

LONDON, NEW YORK, MUNICH,
MELBOURNE, and DELHI

FOR MY STUDENTS

Project Editor Jane Laing
Art Editor Miranda Harvey
Senior Editor Jennifer Jones
Senior Art Editor Karen Sawyer
Managing Editor Gillian Roberts
Category Publisher Mary-Clare Jerram
Art Director Tracy Killick
DTP Designer Louise Waller
Production Controller Wendy Penn

First American edition, 2002
02 03 04 05 10 9 8 7 6 5 4 3 2 1

Published in the United States by
DK Publishing, Inc.
95 Madison Avenue
New York, NY 10016

Library of Congress Cataloging-in-Publication Data
  Meaux, Kia.
    Dynamic yoga / Kia Meaux.
      p. cm.
    Includes index.
    ISBN 0-7894-8064-6 (alk. paper)
    1. Yoga, Hatha. I. Title.

  RA781.7. M42 2002
  613,7'046--dc21   2001055810

Color reproduction by Colourscan, Singapore
Printed and bound in Spain by Artes Graficas Toledo S.A.

See our complete product line at
www.dk.com

CONTENTS

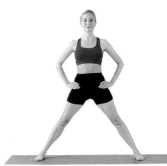
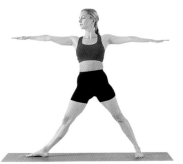
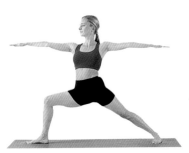

INTRODUCTION

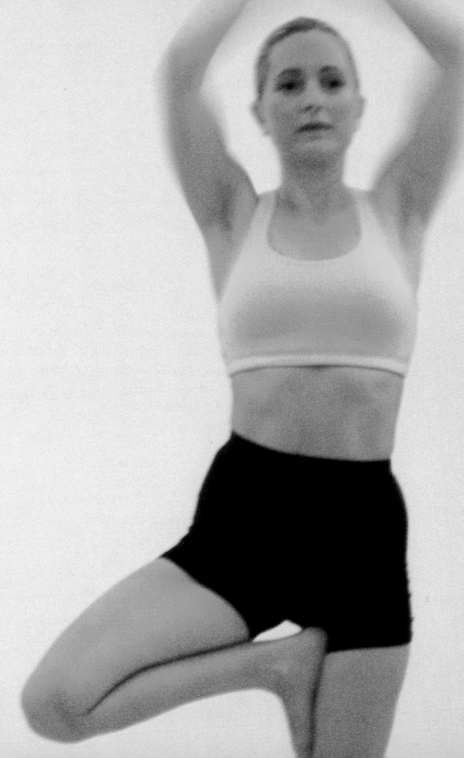

THE DEVELOPMENT OF DYNAMIC YOGA

Dynamic yoga is a creative style of Hatha yoga, blending the principles of Ashtanga and Iyengar. Dynamic yoga is not only meditative but also physically challenging. Central to the technique of dynamic yoga is the sequencing of postures with interlinking transitional movements and a synchronized breathing pattern. These create a flowing connection of yoga postures that gives you a balanced workout and mental clarity.

Yoga is a Sanskrit word that means the union of body, mind, and spirit. Yoga is an exploration of the potential of the body, working in harmony with the mind in order to recognize the higher self. It can be translated as a spiritual union of your soul with God or the eternal truth. This truth is experiential, and the practice of yoga becomes a process of self-discovery that is available to everyone.

Traditionally there are five branches of yoga. They are: Karma yoga – the path of action; Gyana yoga – the path of wisdom; Bhakti yoga – the path of devotion; Hatha yoga – the physical path; and Raja yoga – the path of meditation. The dynamic yoga program in this book is a form of Hatha yoga, which focuses on the physical postures, or *asanas*.

THE BENEFITS OF HATHA YOGA

The practice of yoga involves patience, perseverance, and a keen observation of the self. The consistent practice of yoga postures cultivates the ability to observe what is in the present moment. By focusing your attention on the subtle and broad movements of both mind and body, you are able to gain pure insight into the nature of things as they truly are. This is known as mindfulness, from which follows happiness, freedom, and peace.

The yoga postures demonstrated in this book have been developed from an understanding of the connections between patterns of thought, body posture, and the breath. These connections are evident when you consider the body's habitual response to certain external stimuli. For example, when you are afraid, your heartbeat increases, your breath stops momentarily, and certain muscles tense; when you are nervous, your stomach turns, your breath shortens, and your palms sweat.

Yoga sages have observed these and some more subtle connections between mind and body for thousands of years. Their knowledge is embedded in the dynamic yoga postures. By practicing them, you, too, will reach a deeper understanding of the connections. In time, you will find that you are practicing yoga not only during the movement of postures, but also through the entire day as you go about your regular activities. By bringing the body and mind more in harmony through yoga postures, you will find that your whole approach to life changes. Then, instead of simply reacting to everyday events and situations, you will respond to them mindfully.

This pose is taken from the Sun Salutation A sequence (pp.20–29). The Sun Salutations create the flowing rhythm of the practice.

THE HISTORY OF YOGA

Most of the Hatha yoga forms taught today throughout the Western world are influenced by the great yogi Tirumalai Krishnamacharya, who was born in 1888. He is considered the father of modern yoga and is responsible for pioneering the refinement of postures, specifically sequencing them and giving therapeutic value to each one. He is also responsible for combining the postures with breath control to create a form of moving meditation.

Sri K. Pattabhi Jois, who developed the *Ashtanga Vinyasa* method of Hatha yoga, studied with Krishnamacharya from the age of 12 and continues to teach yoga, inspired by his great teacher, in Mysore, India. B.K.S. Iyengar also studied with Krishnamacharya, albeit for a brief time.

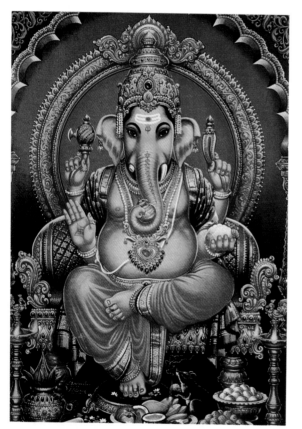

Lord of learning and remover of obstacles, the Hindu god Ganesh provides inspiration to yoga students, who should cultivate the attitude that obstacles are there to be overcome.

He has spent his life perfecting the *asanas* that his first guru taught him and is the founder of the Iyengar style of yoga. He has a yoga center in Pune, India. T. Desikachar, the son of Krishnamacharya, developed the *Viniyoga* approach to Hatha yoga and currently has a yoga center in Chennai, India. He also teaches throughout the world.

THE EIGHT LIMBS

One of the founding principles of Hatha yoga to which dynamic yoga adheres is that of the eight limbs, which is the literal translation of the Sanskrit word *ashtanga*. Devised by the famous sage Patanjali in about 200 B.C., the eight limbs are described by him in the historical yoga text, the *Yoga Sutras.* The eight limbs can be likened to the form and nature of a tree. For, as a tree stands strong against every adversity and continues to grow, producing fruits from its labor, so do yoga students, through consistent practice and dedication, begin to reap the benefits of their labor and nourish the fruits of their love.

The first five limbs are concerned with the body and the brain. They constitute the outer phase of yoga. The final three limbs are concerned with the reconditioning of the mind and constitute the inner phase of yoga.

The first limb of yoga is called *Yama.* Its purpose is to promote moral and ethical principles within the individual. Yama has five principles or social disciplines: *ahimsa* (non-violence), *satya* (truth), *asteya* (non-stealing), *brahmacharya* (purity), and *aparigraha* (non-attachment).

The second limb is called *Niyama.* Its purpose is to create an inner integrity and it also has five principles: *saucha* (cleanliness, purity), *santosha* (contentment), *tapas* (austerity), *svadhaya* (self-study), and *isvarapranidhana* (surrender to God).

The third limb is called *Asana.* These are the yoga postures, which are practiced to calm the mind, enabling a deep state of meditation to occur. This is based on the principle that if the body is restless, the mind will also become restless, inhibiting the true realization of the self.

The fourth limb is *Pranayama,* or extension of the breath. *Prana* is the life-force energy, and *ayama* is the voluntary

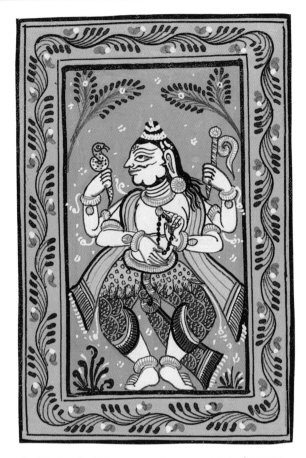

The Hindu deity, Shiva, represents supreme consciousness. He is also known as the Lord of the Dance, symbolizing the eternal movement of the universe.

effort to control and direct this energy. *Pranayama* helps contemplation and eliminates distractions of the mind, so it becomes easier to concentrate and meditate.

The fifth limb is *Pratyahara*, which means mastery of the senses. Through the practice of *asana* and *pranayama* your mind's attention is turned within; through *pratyahara* this internal focus is maintained.

The sixth limb is *Dharana*, or concentration. It is the ability to focus your full attention on one point to the exclusion of everything else. It is essential to realizing the true self.

The seventh limb is *Dhyana*, or meditation, which is the effortless flow of awareness toward the object of concentration. The difference between concentration and

meditation is that in concentration there is a peripheral distraction or awareness of your immediate surroundings, whereas in meditation the attention is not disturbed at all; you are completely absorbed.

The eighth limb is *Samadhi*, which means the absorption of object with the mind. In this enlightened state there is no duality of consciousness. It is one step beyond being completely absorbed in the meditative state. When you have achieved *samadhi*, the "I" becomes nonexistent. You become one with God or one with all. This is the fruit of the tree or the fruits of your labor.

PRACTICING DYNAMIC YOGA

This form of dynamic yoga focuses on the third and fourth limbs of yoga — the *asanas*, or postures, and *pranayama*, or extension of the breath. This book provides a sequence of yoga postures and transition moves that exercises your body and draws your attention to the way the breath can work with the body, helping you to extend it. The transition moves allow you to move your body naturally from one posture to another in a continuous flow, helping you to maintain your concentration and work toward the fifth limb of yoga — *pratyahara*.

The series of dynamic postures and transition moves presented in this book is just one of many possible sequences that can be developed using the interconnecting movements of the Sun Salutations. The entire series will take you at least 90 minutes to complete and offers a very thorough workout of all muscle groups. At the back of the book I have also suggested two shorter programs — one of 60 minutes and one of 30 minutes — that you might like to try if your time is limited. If on any particular day you are very short of time, simply practice the Sun Salutations — both A and B — several times. Remember, five minutes spent practicing dynamic yoga twice a day is more effective than two hours practiced once a week.

Whichever length of program you choose, with regular practice, you will find that not only will your physical body improve, but also your ability to focus and your level of awareness will be enhanced.

BEFORE YOU START

The fundamentals of your dynamic yoga practice are covered here. Correct breath control is essential to creating a seamless flow of postures. Dynamic yoga also draws on the bandhas (inner energy locks) to help extend the breath. This form of yoga is very safe as long as you listen to your body. This in itself may take some practice. Learn to know when your body is out of balance or when you are pushing it too far – and always modify your postures whenever necessary.

BREATH CONTROL

An intrinsic part of the practice of dynamic yoga is the synchronization of the movement of your body with the rhythm of your breathing to energize your body, focus the mind, and avoid muscle strain. Let the sound of your own breath be the music to your dance. Never move unless you are breathing, and synchronize the beginning and end of each breath with the beginning and end of a specific movement. The rhythm of your breath should remain steady and smooth throughout the steps of each posture, which means that you must concentrate on the flow of your breath and take conscious control of your inhalations and exhalations. This is known as *Pranayama*, or breath control. The quality of your breath is an indication of the quality of your practice. If you are holding your breath or it is shallow and strained, you may have gone beyond your limit and should draw back.

In order to stretch your body in the practice of the asanas, you must learn how to stretch, or lengthen, your inhalations and exhalations. *Ujjayi pranayama* is a unique breathing technique that enables you to increase the airflow. It means "victorious extended breath." It involves slightly constricting the glottis (the opening through the vocal chords) as you would if whispering. The friction of the air passing through the constricted glottis has the effect of creating a sound similar to wind moving through a tunnel. The easiest way to begin to cultivate this sound is to lie on your back with the knees bent and feet flat on the floor. Close your eyes, soften your face, and slightly constrict the glottis, keeping your lips together in a hint of

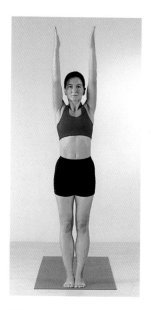

When you are moving the torso or limbs in an upward direction, always inhale.

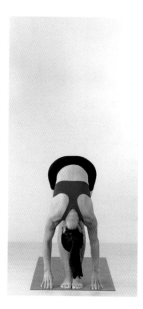

When you are moving the torso or limbs downward, always exhale.

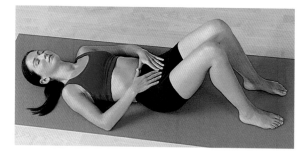

When practicing *Ujjayi pranayama*, rest your thumbs on top of your navel and your fingertips on your lower abdomen. The area beneath your fingertips should not ascend or descend.

a smile. Take deep, long extended breaths without raising and lowering the lower abdomen. Concentrate on moving the breath up, expanding your entire rib cage and the area supporting the kidneys. You should feel your entire back expanding on the floor as you inhale.

The sound can be created by imagining you are saying "haaaaaa" on the exhale and "saaaaaa" on the inhale but keeping the lips together. This sound becomes a tool you can use during your *asana* practice for concentrating your attention. Think of it as your *mantra*. When your mind begins to wander, bring your attention back to the sound and rhythm of your breath.

ALIGNMENT

Correct alignment of the body is crucial when practicing the dynamic yoga postures. The weight of your body must be distributed evenly and grounded in the floor. Checks and balances must be applied, so that the whole body is held in balance for each posture. It is important to sit and stand up straight at the beginning of each posture. By extending the spine, you create more space between the vertebrae, allowing freedom of movement. To support the spine fully, you must engage all the muscles in your body, which you must teach to work in harmony with each other.

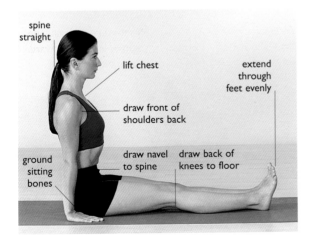

spine straight
lift chest
extend through feet evenly
draw front of shoulders back
ground sitting bones
draw navel to spine
draw back of knees to floor

Dandasana is the starting position for most of the seated poses. Align your shoulders with your wrists and ears, and extend your legs out straight in front of you.

BANDHAS

Bandha is a Sanskrit word that means "lock." By engaging a bandha during an *asana,* you are able to regulate the flow of *prana,* the life-force energy that moves through the body. I have focused on developing two of the three *bandhas* in this dynamic series of poses: *mula bandha* and *uddiyana bandha.*

Mula means "root" in Sanskrit, and you engage *mula bandha* by contracting the perineum, which is located in front of the anus and behind the genitals. The contraction is established toward the end of an exhalation and should be maintained throughout the inhale. To start with, you may notice that you are engaging the entire area, including the anus, but with practice you will be able to refine the action and lift only the perineum.

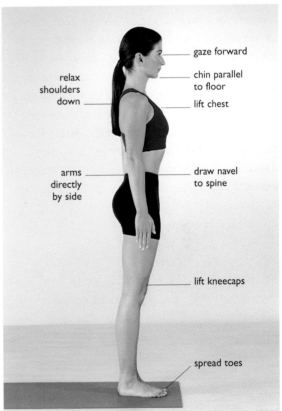

relax shoulders down
gaze forward
chin parallel to floor
lift chest
arms directly by side
draw navel to spine
lift kneecaps
spread toes

Tadasana is the starting position for most of the standing poses. Bring your head back, so that your ears, shoulders, and hips are all aligned. Look straight ahead.

The second bandha is called *uddiyana*, which means "flying upward." This lock is engaged by drawing in the abdominal wall (just a few inches below the navel and above the pubic bone). It is a very subtle drawing of the back of the navel to the spine, which allows your lower abdomen to remain soft and still. This lift is connected with the drawing up of the perineum and will also be most apparent at the end of an exhalation. You can practice both of these energy locks in the Downward Dog (*Adho mukha svanasana*) position in the Sun Salutation sequences. Notice that both *mula bandha* and *uddiyana bandha* connect with the breath. Have patience: the engagement of the *bandhas* takes years to master fully and you will learn to engage them only with practice.

HOW TO PRACTICE

Do not practice dynamic yoga on a full stomach. It is best to wait two to three hours after eating before beginning a program. Choose a time in the day when you will not be interrupted or distracted: you need to be able to give your full attention to practicing the *asanas*. It is important to be comfortable, and the clothing you wear when doing dynamic yoga must be flexible and able to breath. The fabrics that work best are cotton blend.

Practice in a quiet, clean, warm environment. A wooden floor is ideal, and the perfect floor is one that allows you to practice without a "sticky mat." However, if the surface of your floor is slippery, you must use a mat.

Avoid vigorous practice while menstruating, as this can disrupt the flow of menses. Instead, I suggest practicing *Utthita trikonasana* (*pp.48–49*), *Baddha konasana* (*pp.128–129*), and *Balasana* (*p.135*), all of which are soothing and can help relieve cramping. It is very important at this time to avoid all inverted poses (upside-down poses). Ideally, you should ask a dynamic yoga teacher to advise on the specific practice you can do while menstruating.

MODIFICATIONS

It is important not to push your body beyond its limits when practicing dynamic yoga. If you find that a particular posture creates strain or tension in a part of your body, withdraw from it. A pose done with force can be very injurious, and usually results in undue pressure being applied to another area of the body to compensate.

In many cases in this book, a specific, less strenuous, alternative is shown. For example, if you cannot reach the floor with your left arm in *Parivrtta parsvakonasana* (*pp.60–61*), then bend your arms into prayer position as shown in the alternative. If no alternative is shown, there are two modifications of body position that between them can be applied to most postures. The first is simply to bend

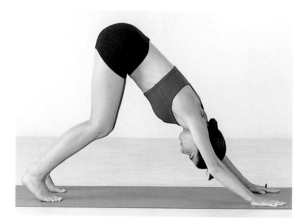

If you have tight hips and hamstrings and it is difficult for you to straighten the spine, the best option is to bend the knees, allowing the spine to lengthen.

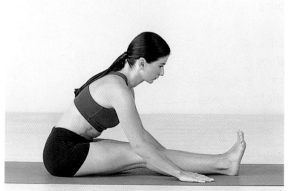

If you find that you cannot reach your toes when you fold forward while sitting, then rather than allowing your spine to curve forward, reach less far forward with your arms.

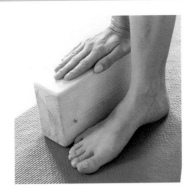

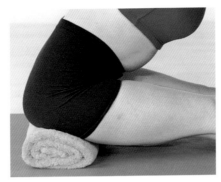

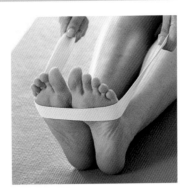

Place a block next to your foot and rest your hand on it if you cannot reach the floor without straining.

A rolled-up towel placed beneath your sitting bones will allow you to fold your body farther forward.

Wrapping a strap around your feet will allow you to deepen a forward bend without applying force.

your legs where the full pose calls for straight legs. The second is to keep your legs straight but to reach less far forward with your arms. You can gradually move your body toward the full pose as you practice.

In addition to modifying the position of your body to avoid straining, you can also use equipment to help you in positions that cause difficulty. For example, blocks can be very useful in helping you to balance in the standing poses if you cannot reach the floor with your hand. Equally, if your hips are tight and restrict you as you fold forward, a rolled towel or blanket placed under the sitting bones will help, and will also mean that you do not harm the lower back. If you cannot reach your toes with your hands, try using a strap to enable you to deepen the stretch.

SPECIAL CIRCUMSTANCES

If you have a specific injury or known weakness, then you must be very careful not to place any strain on that area of the body when practicing yoga. For example, if you have a neck injury, avoid postures that require you to roll onto it, such as *Sarvangasana* (pp.136–137), without the guidance of a qualified teacher. It is equally important to be careful if you have a back injury or strain. It is best to practice with a teacher until you understand the appropriate alternatives for your particular injury. Something as common as tight hips can be helped by using a towel or modifying your position. For tight hamstrings, bend the legs when you

cannot straighten them, and pay particular attention to the symmetry and alignment of your legs in each posture.

If you are pregnant, it is best not to practice dynamic yoga. There are yoga classes tailored especially for pregnant women; try one of these for this period. You can come back to dynamic yoga after the birth and when your doctor gives you clearance.

RESTING

It is very important to rest when necessary and not to push yourself to a state of exhaustion. If you need to rest between postures, rest in *Balasana* (p.135). At the end of each program rest in *Savasana* (p.144), using this pose to farther your ability to meditate.

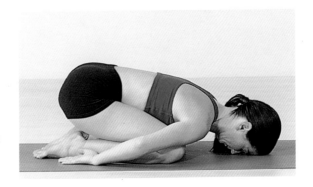

Balasana, or Child's pose, is particularly good for releasing tension in the shoulders and neck, making it an ideal posture to go into after *Sirsasana*. Use it whenever you need to rest.

WARMING UP

It is best to spend a few minutes gently stretching before performing the sun salutations. Most of us tend to spend hours just sitting, creating tightness in the hips and often putting a strain on the spine. Doing two of the four warm-up exercises presented here before beginning a dynamic yoga program helps release any stiffness in the back and shoulders. This prepares the body for the relative intensity of the Sun Salutation sequences.

Happy Pose

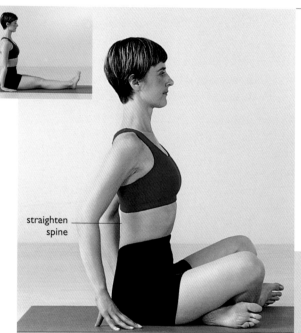

straighten spine

1 Sit on the floor with your legs out straight in front of you and your arms straight by your sides. Inhaling, cross the right leg over the left. Move your hands back slightly and bend your arms, pressing down with your fingertips to straighten the spine. Gaze forward.

2 Exhaling, fold the body forward, reaching out with your arms. Hold for two to five minutes, breathing slowly. With each inhale lengthen the spine and with each exhale deepen the fold in the hips. Repeat with the left leg crossed over the right.

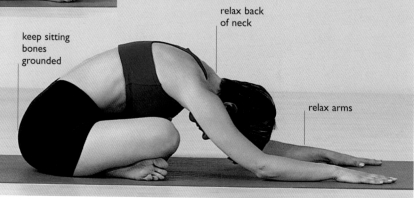

keep sitting bones grounded

relax back of neck

relax arms

Wide Butterfly

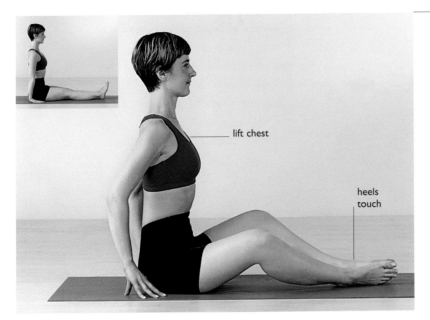

lift chest

heels touch

1 Sit in the same position as for Happy Pose. Inhaling, bring the heels of your feet together, bending your legs slightly. Let your knees fall out to the sides. Move your hands back slightly and press down with your fingertips.

2 Exhaling, fold the body forward from the hips, grounding the sitting bones and reaching out with your arms. Let your whole body relax over the legs. Hold for two to five minutes.

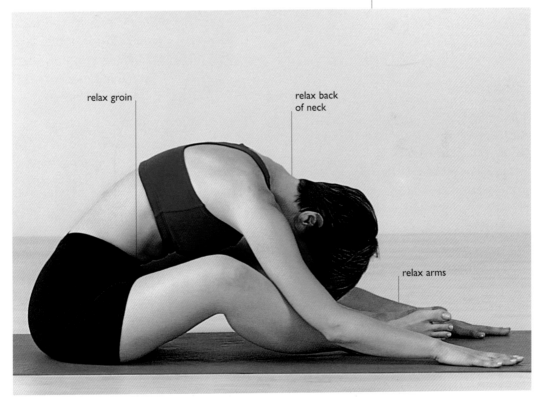

relax groin

relax back of neck

relax arms

Spinal Roll

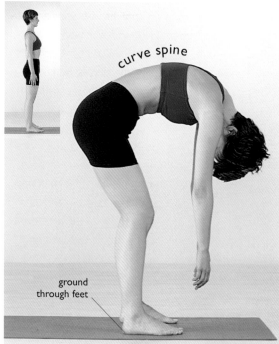

curve spine

ground through feet

1 Stand up straight with your arms by your sides, feet hip-width apart, and toes spread. Exhaling, bend at the knees and fold your body forward slowly, letting the weight of the upper body take the torso forward. Allow the spine to curve and the arms to hang down.

2 Continue exhaling until the hands are touching the floor and the entire torso is flopping forward. Relax the back of the neck and let the weight of the head pull the neck long. Hold the pose for 10 breaths. Then, inhaling, roll the body up to standing.

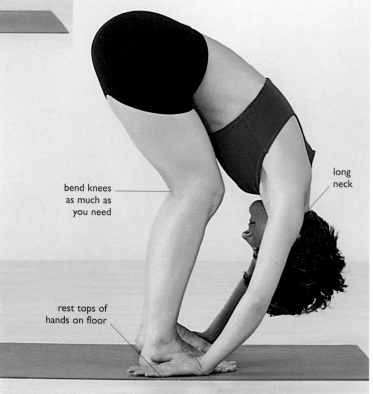

bend knees as much as you need

long neck

rest tops of hands on floor

Arms Wrapped Forward Bend

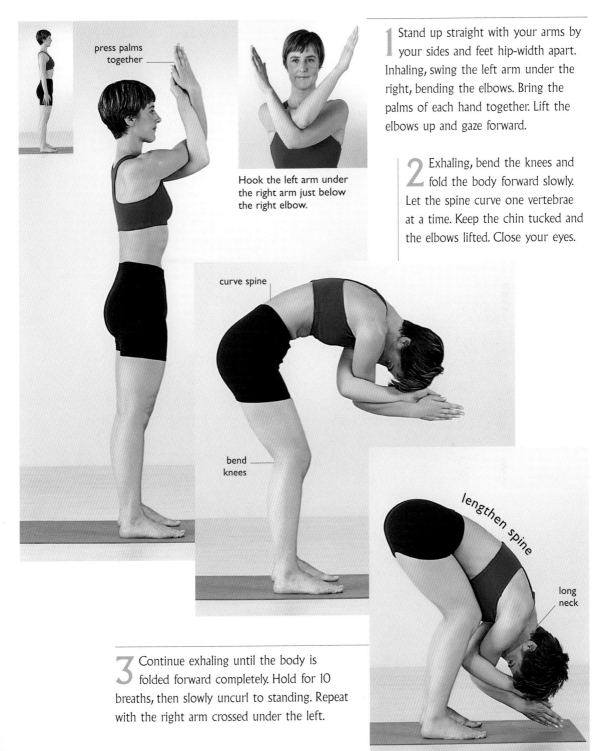

press palms together

Hook the left arm under the right arm just below the right elbow.

curve spine

bend knees

lengthen spine

long neck

1 Stand up straight with your arms by your sides and feet hip-width apart. Inhaling, swing the left arm under the right, bending the elbows. Bring the palms of each hand together. Lift the elbows up and gaze forward.

2 Exhaling, bend the knees and fold the body forward slowly. Let the spine curve one vertebrae at a time. Keep the chin tucked and the elbows lifted. Close your eyes.

3 Continue exhaling until the body is folded forward completely. Hold for 10 breaths, then slowly uncurl to standing. Repeat with the right arm crossed under the left.

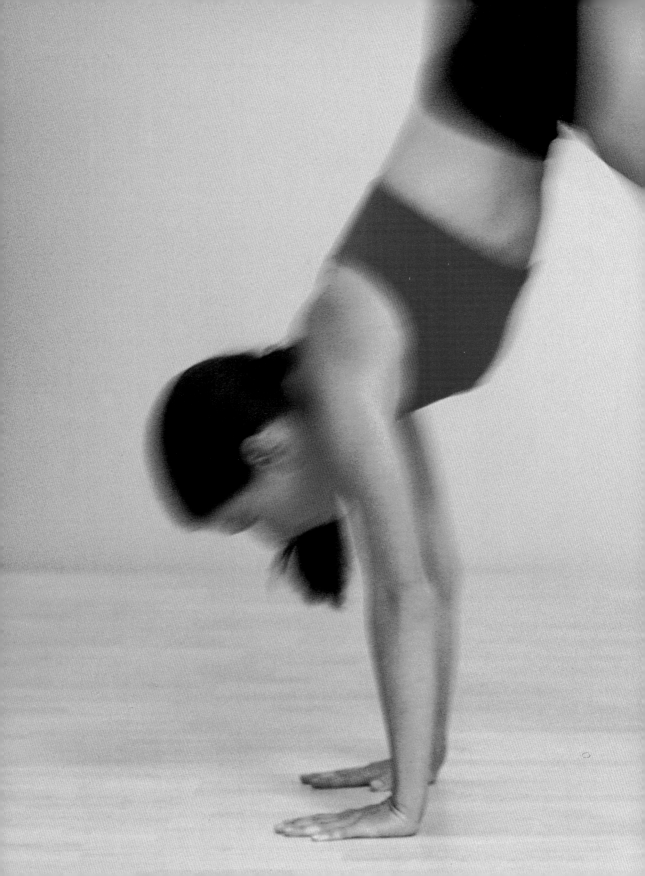

THE SUN
SALUTATIONS

SURYA NAMASKARA A
Sun Salutation A

The Sun Salutation sequences warm up the body and draw the attention to the rhythm of the breath. Each movement is synchronized to an inhalation or exhalation. Sun Salutation A builds up muscular strength and is particularly important for strengthening the cardiovascular and respiratory systems. It can also alleviate depression and anxiety.

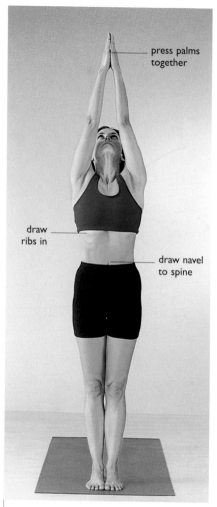

press palms together

draw ribs in

draw navel to spine

1 **Tadasana** Stand tall, your feet together, arms by your sides. Distribute your weight equally across the soles of your feet and spread the toes evenly. Exhaling, draw the lower belly in and up, and raise the center of the perineum as you lift the core of your body, bringing awareness to *mula bandha*. Gaze straight ahead.

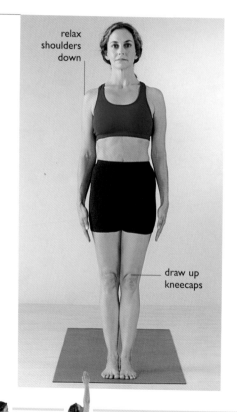

relax shoulders down

draw up kneecaps

2 **Raised Tadasana** Inhaling, sweep your arms out to the sides of the body and raise them high above your head. Press your palms together at the end of the breath. Look up at your thumbs.

whole sequence at a glance

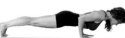

Exhaling.......Inhaling......Exhaling.........Inhaling.................Exhaling.............

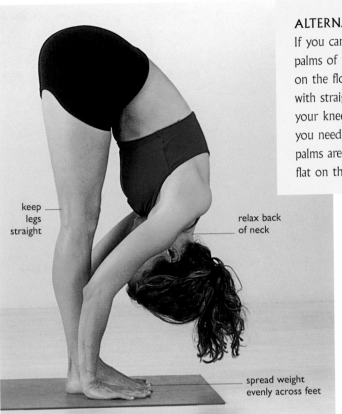

keep legs straight

relax back of neck

spread weight evenly across feet

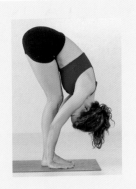

ALTERNATIVE
If you cannot place the palms of your hands flat on the floor by your feet with straight legs, bend your knees as much as you need until your palms are completely flat on the floor.

3 Uttanasana Exhaling, pull back the pubic bone and fold your body forward. Place your hands flat on the floor either side of, and parallel to, your feet. At the end of the exhale, gaze at your navel.

4 Ardha Uttanasana Inhaling, look up, lifting the torso halfway up. Straighten the spine and pull back the pubic bone. Straighten your arms and place your fingertips on the floor. Gaze slightly forward.

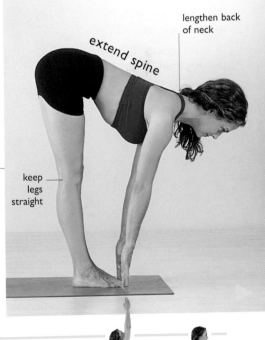

lengthen back of neck

extend spine

keep legs straight

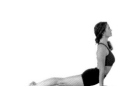 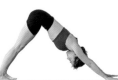 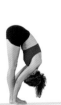 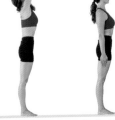

..........Inhaling.................Exhaling...............Inhaling..........Exhaling......Inhaling......Exhaling

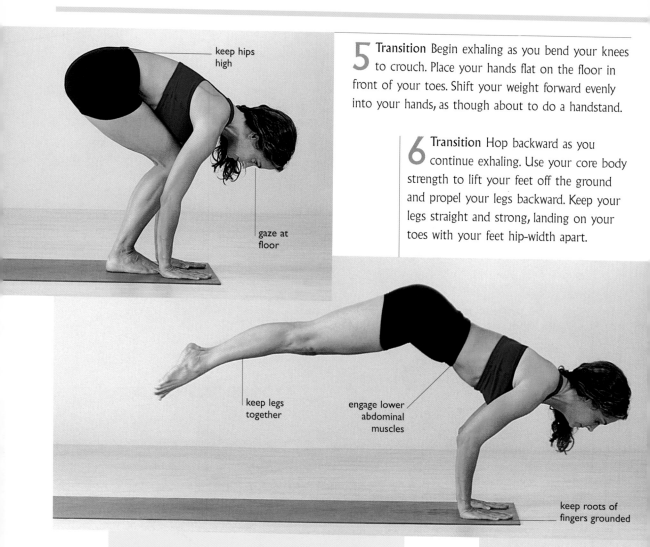

keep hips high

gaze at floor

5 **Transition** Begin exhaling as you bend your knees to crouch. Place your hands flat on the floor in front of your toes. Shift your weight forward evenly into your hands, as though about to do a handstand.

6 **Transition** Hop backward as you continue exhaling. Use your core body strength to lift your feet off the ground and propel your legs backward. Keep your legs straight and strong, landing on your toes with your feet hip-width apart.

keep legs together

engage lower abdominal muscles

keep roots of fingers grounded

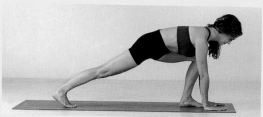

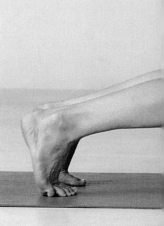

ALTERNATIVE
If jumping back is difficult, try stepping back into the push-up position. Keep your hands flat on the floor and arms straight. Step the right and then the left foot back, placing the feet hip-width apart.

ALTERNATIVE

If you are unable to perform *Chaturanga* without strain, place your knees on the ground and then lower the rest of your body toward the floor. Keep your elbows close in to your torso and directly above your wrists. Gaze down. Practice this to build up your arm strength.

7 Chaturanga Dhandasana
Exhaling, fully engage your muscles and lower your body evenly until it is 4–6in (10–15cm) above, and parallel to, the floor in the push-up position. Keep your bent elbows in very close to your sides and directly above your wrists. Gaze down.

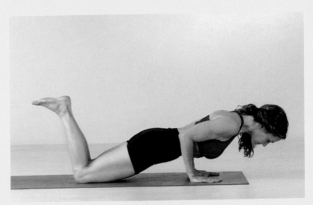

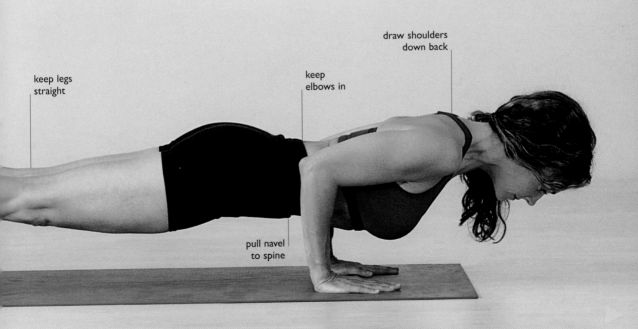

keep legs straight

keep elbows in

draw shoulders down back

pull navel to spine

ALTERNATIVE

If you are unable to push your whole body off the floor, lift only the chest and rib cage, keeping the belly and pubic bone on the floor. Keep your arms bent, but make sure your fingertips align with the tops of the shoulders and your elbows are held close to your body.

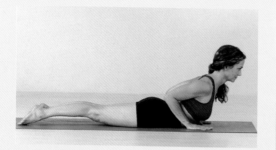

8 **Urdhva Mukha Svanasana** Inhaling, push off the balls of your feet, rolling your feet forward over the tips of your toes. Straighten your arms and pull your hips forward. Lift your chest up so that your whole body is raised completely off the floor. Point your toes and gaze straight ahead.

Roll your feet over the tips of your toes until the tops of your feet rest on the floor.

keep legs straight and firm

arch back

allow belly to stretch

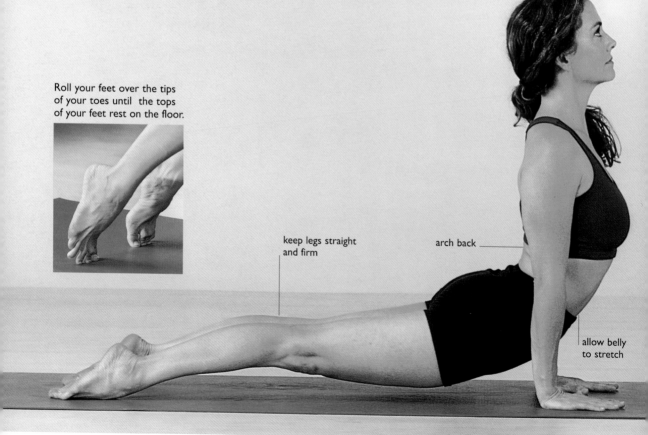

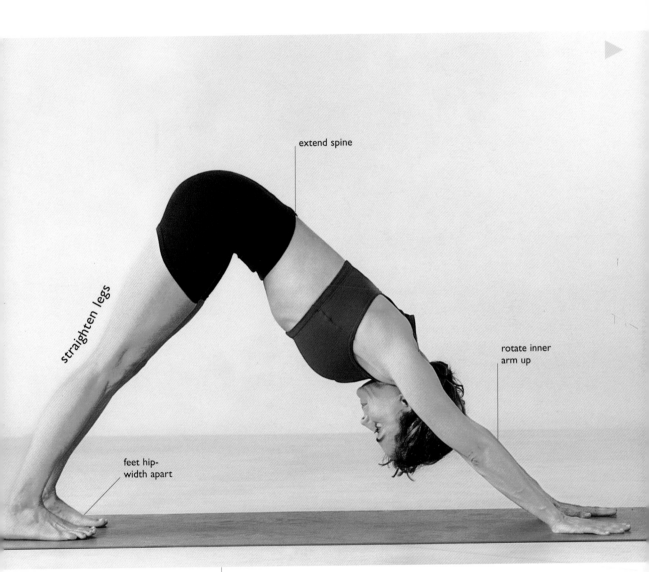

extend spine

straighten legs

rotate inner arm up

feet hip-
width apart

9 **Adho Mukha Svanasana** Exhaling, push your hips up, rolling back over your toes and lowering the heels onto the floor. If you cannot set your feet flat on the floor, bend the knees slightly and let the heels lift off as much as you need. Spread out your fingers and lift the sitting bones up toward the ceiling. Stretch out your arms, lift the kneecaps, and firm the muscles at the front of your thighs. Gaze at the navel.

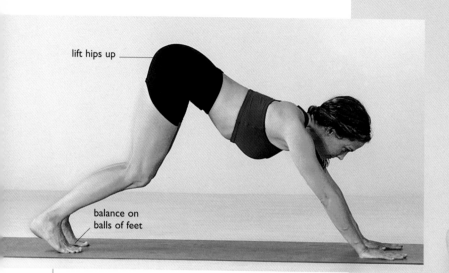

lift hips up

balance on
balls of feet

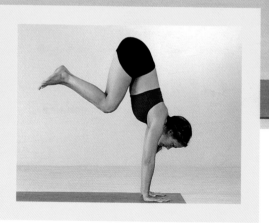

keep legs straight

10 **Transition** Prepare to hop forward. Begin exhaling as you bend your knees and look forward between the hands. Move all of your weight into the hands as though you were going to do a handstand. Lift the hips up high, ready to push off on the balls of your feet.

ALTERNATIVE
If you find it difficult keeping your legs straight when hopping forward, hop forward with your legs bent. As you push off your feet, the weight of your body shifts to the hands, rooting the fingers to the floor. Keep your hips high and look down between your hands.

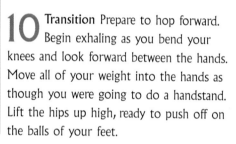

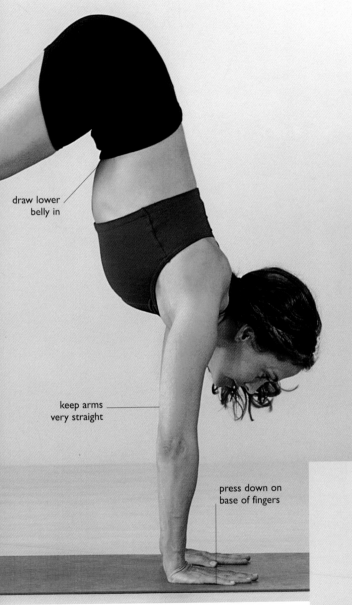

draw lower
belly in

keep arms
very straight

press down on
base of fingers

11 **Transition** Continue exhaling as you hop forward. Push off the feet and straighten the legs, keeping the hips high in the air. Engage both *uddiyana* and *mula bandha* to lift the torso. Keep your arms straight and shoulder-width apart. Gaze down between the hands.

12 **Transition** At the end of the exhale, land in a crouch with your feet together and between your hands. Keep your palms flat on the floor throughout the move. Gaze down.

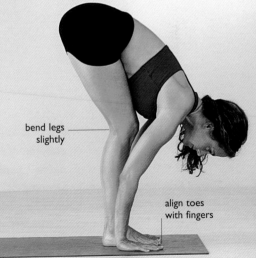

bend legs
slightly

align toes
with fingers

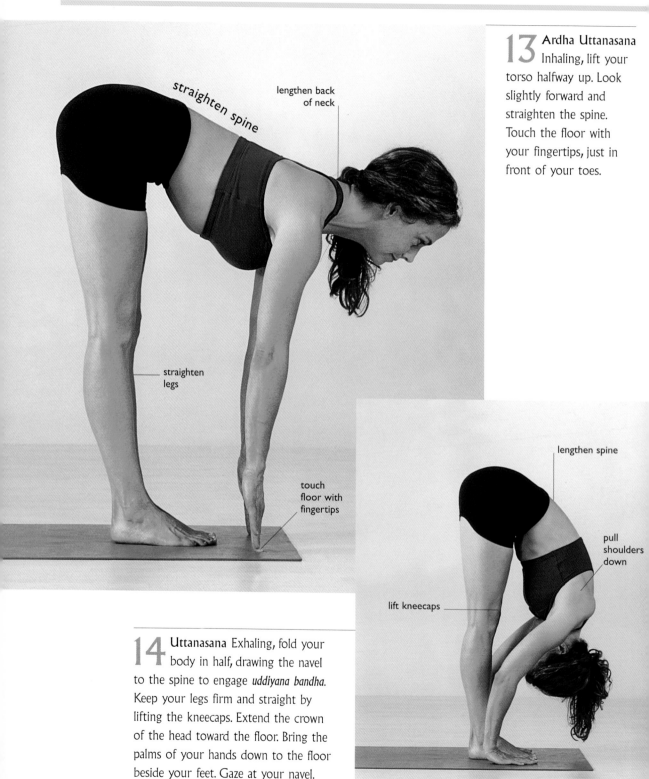

straighten spine

lengthen back
of neck

straighten
legs

touch
floor with
fingertips

13 **Ardha Uttanasana**
Inhaling, lift your
torso halfway up. Look
slightly forward and
straighten the spine.
Touch the floor with
your fingertips, just in
front of your toes.

lengthen spine

pull
shoulders
down

lift kneecaps

14 **Uttanasana** Exhaling, fold your
body in half, drawing the navel
to the spine to engage *uddiyana bandha*.
Keep your legs firm and straight by
lifting the kneecaps. Extend the crown
of the head toward the floor. Bring the
palms of your hands down to the floor
beside your feet. Gaze at your navel.

15 Raised Tadasana Inhaling, sweep your arms out to the side and up, bringing the palms together above your head. Gaze up toward the thumbs. Lengthen the waist without hunching the shoulders.

16 Tadasana Exhaling, sweep your arms back out to the sides and down straight close to the body, palms inward. Standing tall, extend through the crown of the head. Face forward.

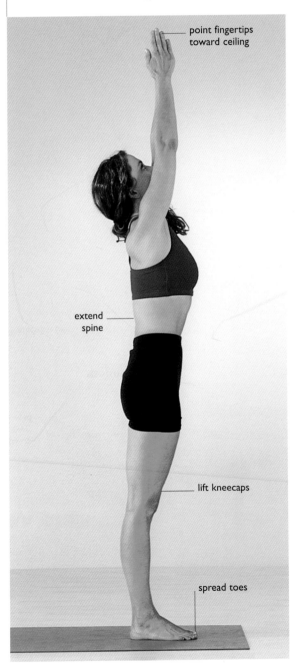

point fingertips toward ceiling

extend spine

lift kneecaps

spread toes

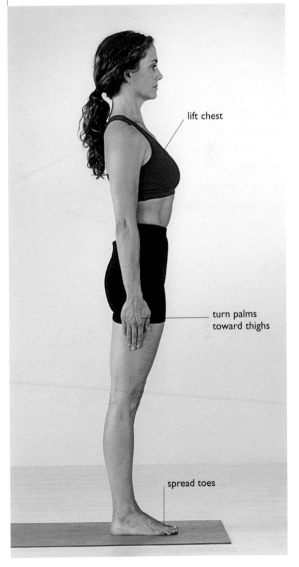

lift chest

turn palms toward thighs

spread toes

SURYA NAMASKARA B
Sun Salutation B

A longer sequence of movements than Sun Salutation A, Sun Salutation B farther strengthens the cardiovascular and respiratory systems, stretching the breath and building up heat within your body. The transitional moves between the new postures are particularly demanding. When you have completed the sequence, repeat, leading with the other leg.

1 Tadasana Stand tall, your feet together, arms by your sides. Distribute your weight equally across the soles of your feet and spread the toes evenly. Exhaling, draw the lower belly in and up, while raising the center of the perineum, bringing awareness to *mula bandha.* Gaze straight ahead.

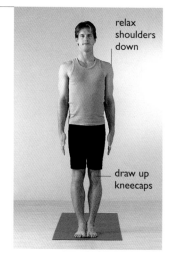

relax shoulders down

draw up kneecaps

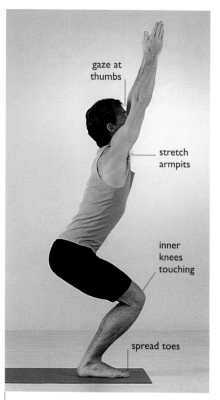

gaze at thumbs

stretch armpits

inner knees touching

spread toes

2 Utkatasana Inhaling, reach up with your arms and press your palms together. Bend your knees and draw back the lower belly and sitting bones into a standing squat.

whole sequence at a glance

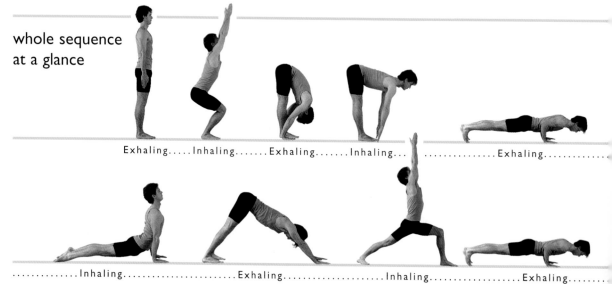

Exhaling.....Inhaling.......Exhaling.......Inhaling... ....Exhaling.............

..........Inhaling...................Exhaling...................Inhaling.................Exhaling........

3 **Uttanasana** Exhaling, fold your body forward, drawing back the pubic bone and bending at the hips. Bring your arms down and place your palms on the floor beside your feet. Let your head hang down, and gaze at your navel or between your legs.

4 **Ardha Uttanasana** Inhaling, lift your torso, keeping your spine straight and your leg muscles engaged. Straighten your arms, touching the floor in front of your toes with your fingertips. Look at the floor slightly in front.

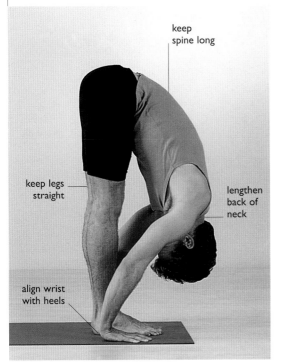

keep spine long

keep legs straight

lengthen back of neck

align wrist with heels

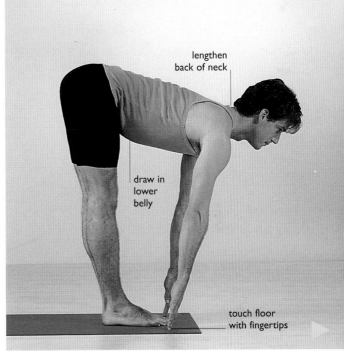

lengthen back of neck

draw in lower belly

touch floor with fingertips

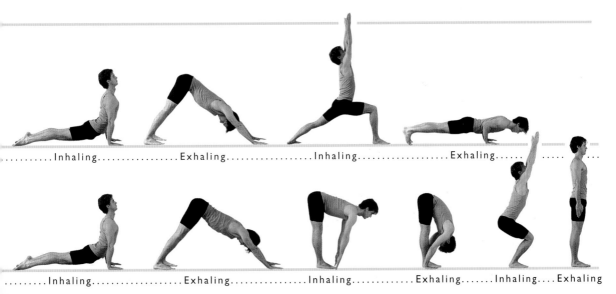

.........Inhaling..................Exhaling..................Inhaling..................Exhaling.............

.........Inhaling..................Exhaling..................Inhaling.............Exhaling.......Inhaling....Exhaling

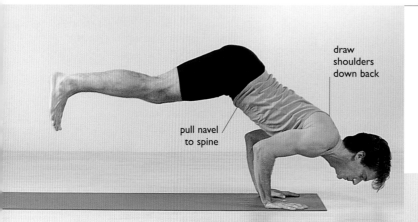

draw
shoulders
down back

pull navel
to spine

5 **Transition** Exhaling, shift your
weight forward onto the hands
and bend your arms. Engaging *mula*
and *uddiyana bandha,* raise your hips
in the air and propel the legs
backward. Land with your feet hip-
width apart. Look down at the floor.

6 **Chaturanga**
Dhandasana Exhaling,
lower your body 4–6in
(10–15cm) above the floor
and parallel to it in the
push-up position. Keep
your shoulders square and
elbows close to the body.
Gaze down at the floor.

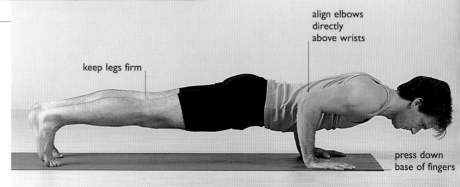

align elbows
directly
above wrists

keep legs firm

press down
base of fingers

7 **Urdhva Mukha**
Svanasana Inhaling,
roll forward over your
toes, so the tops of your
feet are resting on the
floor (*see p.24*). Straighten
your arms and pull your
hips forward, arching your
spine and stretching the
belly. Gaze slightly upward.

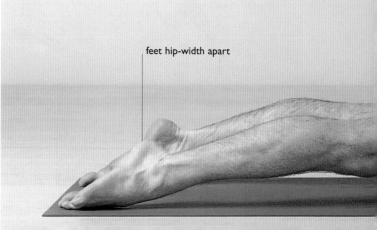

feet hip-width apart

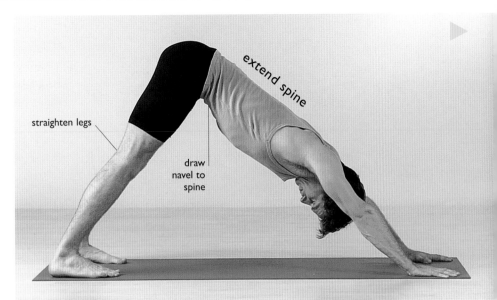

straighten legs

extend spine

draw
navel to
spine

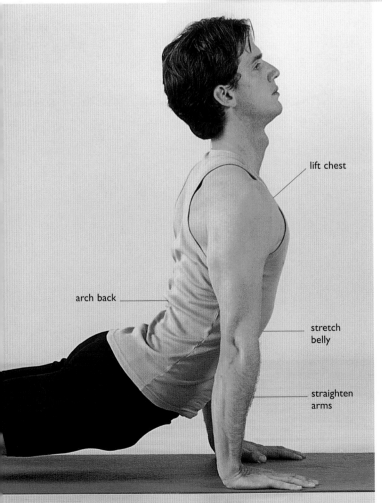

lift chest

arch back

stretch
belly

straighten
arms

8 **Adho Mukha Svanasana** Exhaling, roll back over your toes and pull back the pubic bone as you lower your heels toward the floor. Do not change the position of your hands or feet. Push your hips up in the air, stretch the spine long, and press away from the floor with the base of your fingers. Tuck in your chin very slightly, and gaze at your navel.

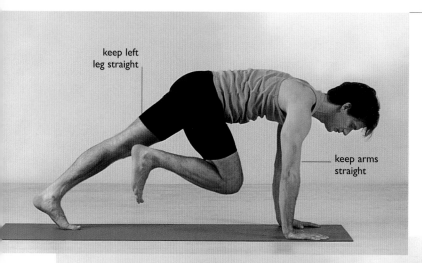

keep left
leg straight

keep arms
straight

9 **Transition** Begin
inhaling as you step
forward with your right
foot. Make sure your right
knee is also facing forward.
Move forward onto the ball
of your left foot. Gaze down
between your hands.

align knee
with ankle

10 **Transition**
Continue inhaling
as you place your right
foot between your hands
and parallel to them.
Make sure the knee is
directly over the ankle.
Raise your head to gaze
slightly forward.

lift sternum

11 **Transition** As you
continue inhaling,
turn your left heel in
about 45° and place the
left foot flat on the floor.
Sweep your arms out to
the sides, turning the
palms up. Gaze ahead.

12 **Virabhadrasana A** At the end of the inhale, bring your palms together above your head, extend through the fingertips, and lengthen the torso. Keep your right knee directly over the ankle. Draw in the ribs to prevent the lower back from arching. Lift the center of the perineum, engaging *mula bandha.* Gaze at the thumbs.

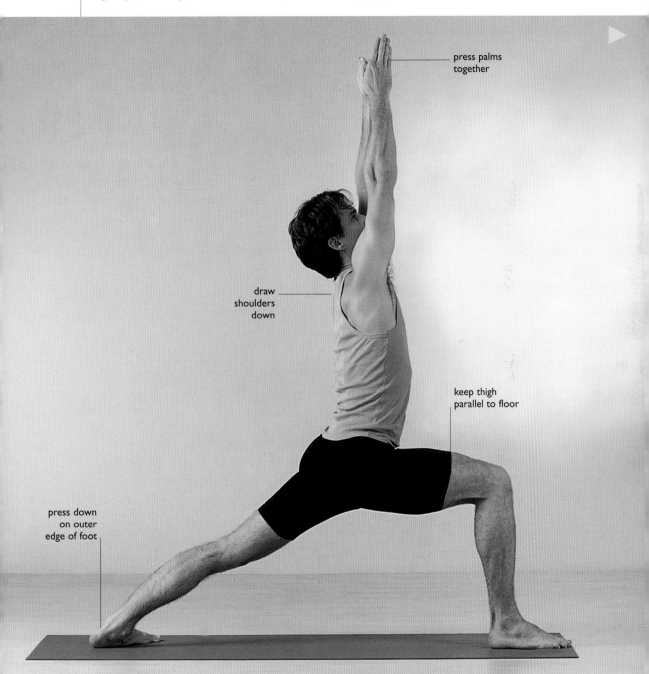

press palms together

draw shoulders down

keep thigh parallel to floor

press down on outer edge of foot

13 **Transition** Begin exhaling as you move your arms out and down toward the floor. Place your hands directly below your shoulders, palms flat on the floor. Lift the heel of your left foot and gaze down and slightly forward. Step back with your right foot so it is parallel with the left.

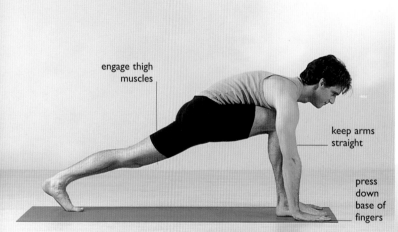

engage thigh muscles

keep arms straight

press down base of fingers

14 **Chaturanga Dhandasana** Exhaling, lower your body 4–6in (10–15cm) above the floor and parallel to it. Keep your shoulders square and elbows close to the body. Gaze down at the floor.

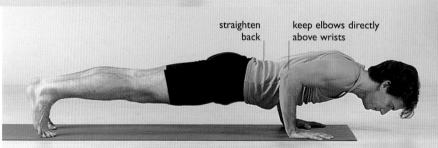

straighten back

keep elbows directly above wrists

15 **Urdhva Mukha Svanasana** Inhaling, pull your hips forward and roll forward over your toes (*see p.24*). Arch your spine and stretch the belly. Gaze slightly upward.

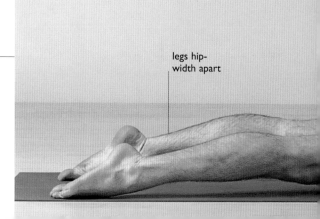

legs hip-width apart

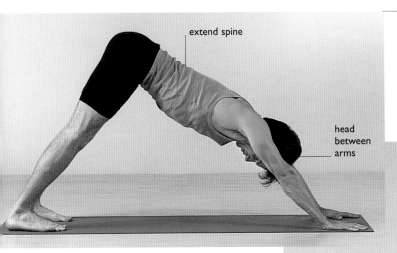

extend spine

head between arms

16 **Adho Mukha Svanasana** Exhaling, roll back over your toes and raise your hips as you lower your heels toward the floor. Press away from the floor with the roots of your fingers.

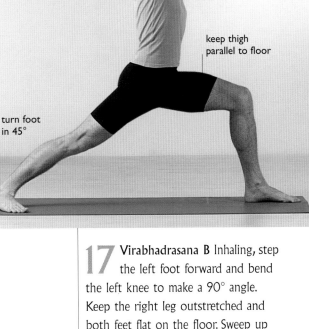

gaze up at thumbs

lengthen torso

keep thigh parallel to floor

turn foot in 45°

17 **Virabhadrasana B** Inhaling, step the left foot forward and bend the left knee to make a 90° angle. Keep the right leg outstretched and both feet flat on the floor. Sweep up with your arms and press your palms together. Gaze up at your thumbs.

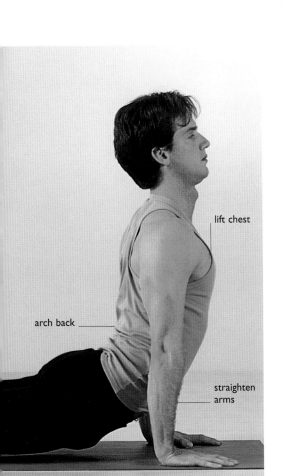

lift chest

arch back

straighten arms

18 Chaturanga Dhandasana Exhaling, sweep your arms out and down toward the floor. Place your hands directly below your shoulders. Step back with your left foot and lower your body so it is parallel to the floor, keeping your legs firm and straight. Draw your navel to the spine and gaze at the floor.

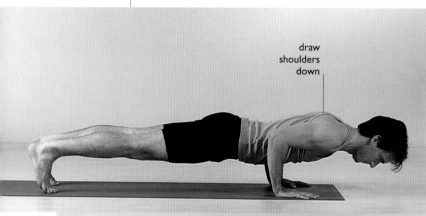

draw
shoulders
down

19 Urdhva Mukha Svanasana Inhaling, roll forward over your toes so the tops of your feet are resting on the floor (*see p.24*). Straighten your arms, lift your chest, and arch your spine. Gaze ahead and slightly upward.

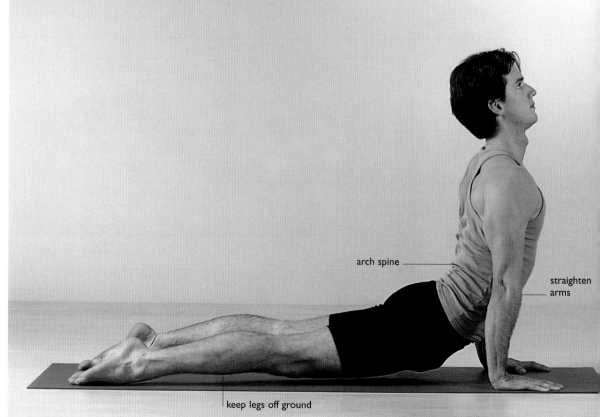

arch spine

straighten arms

keep legs off ground

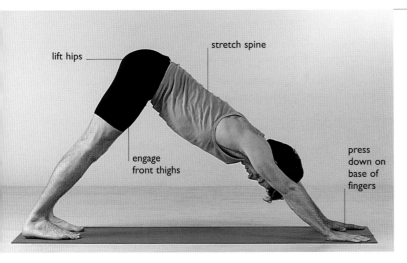

lift hips

stretch spine

engage
front thighs

press
down on
base of
fingers

20 **Adho Mukha Svanasana**
Exhaling, roll over your
toes onto the soles of your feet,
pressing the heels to the floor. Lift
your hips high toward the ceiling
and draw back the pubic bone.
Extend your spine long. Gaze at
your navel.

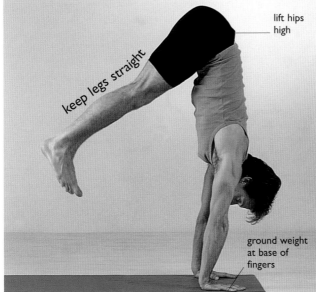

lift hips
high

keep legs straight

ground weight
at base of
fingers

21 **Transition** Exhaling, hop
forward. Push off your feet
with legs slightly bent and raise your
hips high in the air, engaging both
mula and *uddiyana bandha.* Straighten
your legs in a pike and bring them
in toward your body. Keep your arms
straight. Gaze at the floor.

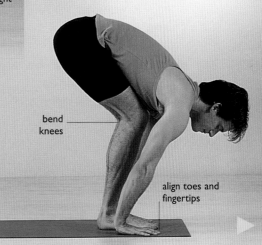

bend
knees

align toes and
fingertips

22 **Transition** At the end of
the exhale, land with both
feet together between your hands.
Bend your knees slightly as you land
in a crouch position. Distribute your
weight equally throughout your
hands and feet.

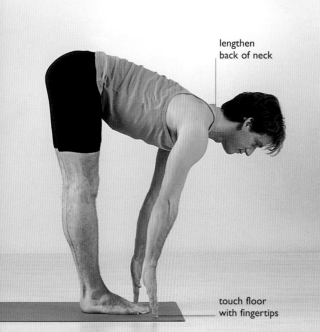

lengthen
back of neck

touch floor
with fingertips

23 **Ardha Uttanasana** Inhaling, lift your sternum and straighten your spine. Straighten your arms, touching the floor in front of your toes with your fingertips. Keep your kneecaps lifted. Gaze at the floor ahead.

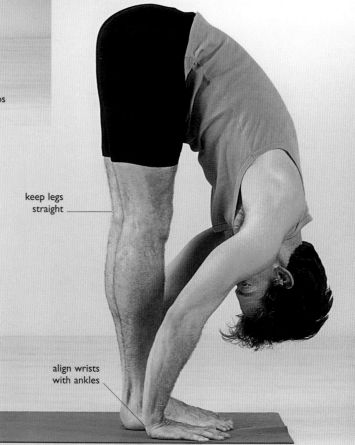

keep legs
straight

align wrists
with ankles

24 **Uttanasana** Exhaling, fold the body forward from the hips, lengthening the spine all the way down. Reach for the floor with the crown of your head and place your palms flat on the floor beside, and parallel to, your feet. Gaze at your navel.

25 **Utkatasana** Inhaling, sweep your arms out to the sides and raise them above your head. Bend your knees and draw back the lower belly and sitting bones into a standing squat. Bring your palms together at the end of the breath.

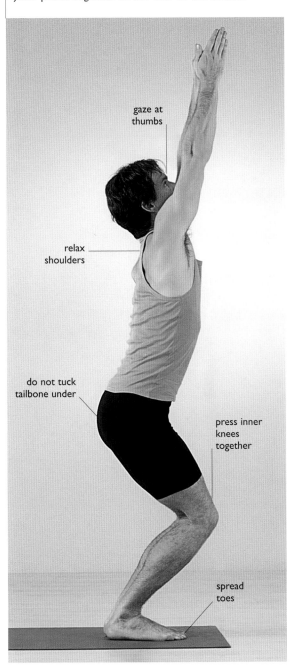

gaze at thumbs

relax shoulders

do not tuck tailbone under

press inner knees together

spread toes

26 **Tadasana** Exhaling, straighten your legs and lower your arms by your side, palms inward. Stand very tall and lengthen the entire body. Gaze forward.

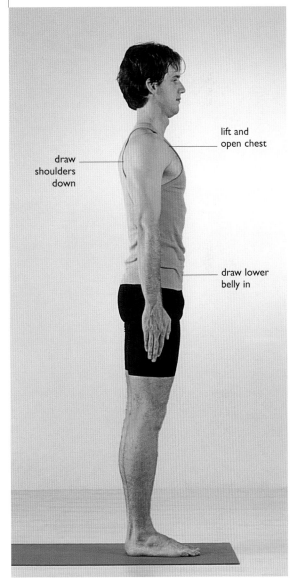

lift and open chest

draw shoulders down

draw lower belly in

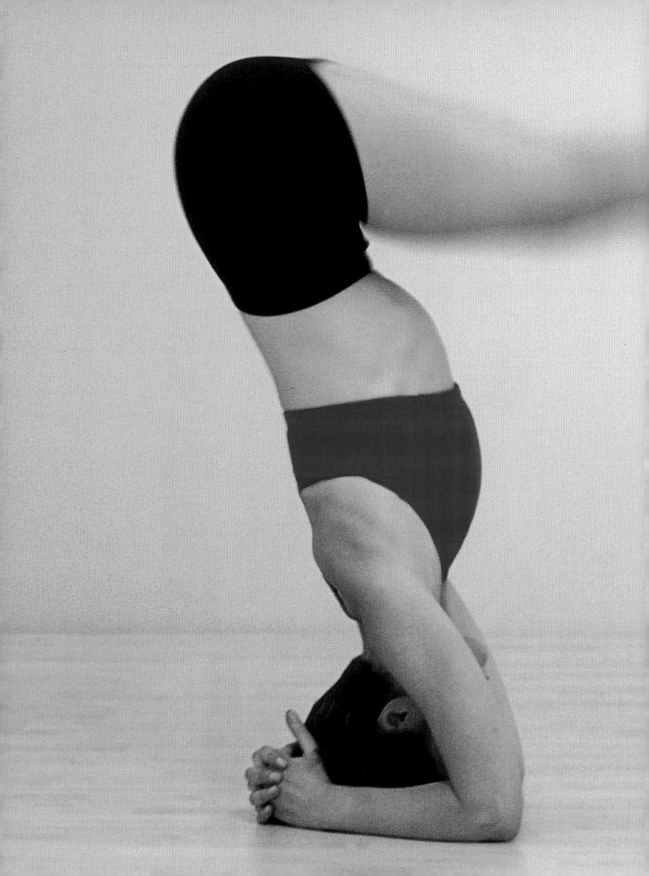

THE
PRACTICE

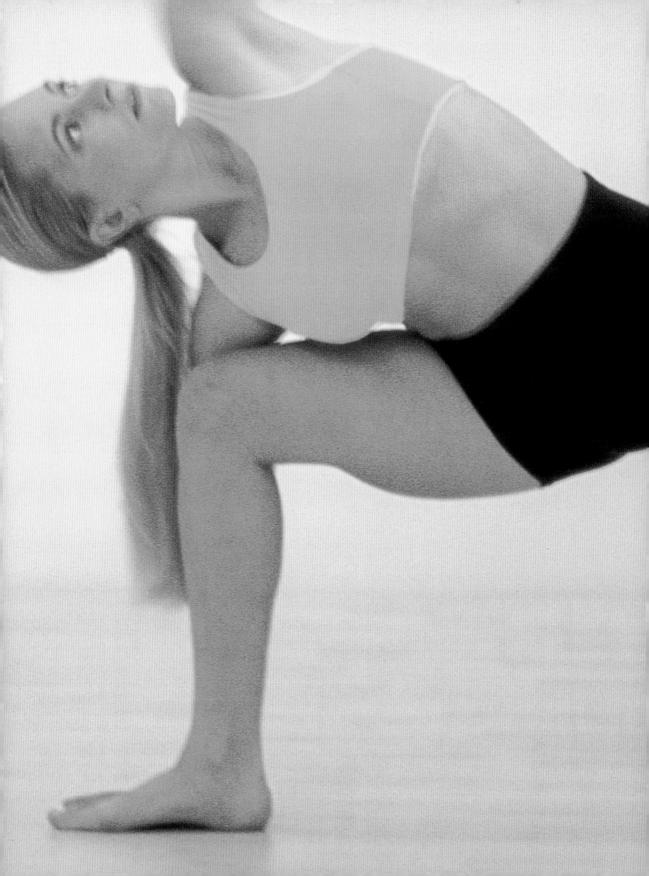

STANDING POSES

Now that you have warmed up the body adequately and aligned your breath, it is time to begin the standing postures. With this selection of standing *asanas*, you will learn balance and the importance of alignment. Be patient: with practice and application you will soon notice an improvement in your physical ability and mental focus.

TRANSITION MOVE
Jumping Out to the Side

Jumping is a transitional movement you can use after completing the Sun Salutations and also, if you wish, between the standing poses shown on pages 48 to 67. It is an exhilarating move and excellent for developing stamina and coordination. Do not jump if you suffer from back or knee problems, or during menstruation. In these cases it is better simply to step out and back.

1 Stand at the front of the mat with your feet together. Bring your hands together in the prayer position in front of your chest. Exhaling, squat down and prepare to jump. Hold your weight slightly forward. Gaze ahead.

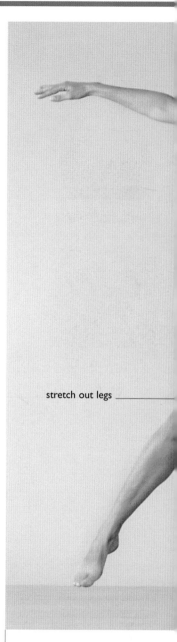

stretch out legs _____

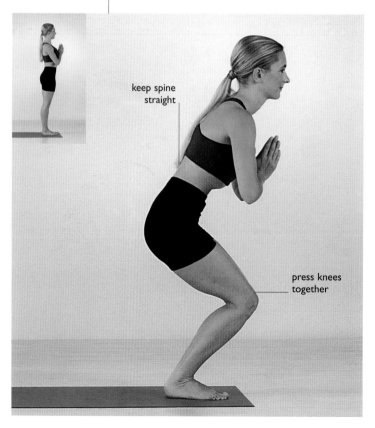

keep spine
straight

press knees
together

2 Inhaling, jump, spreading your arms out wide. Lift both feet off the floor simultaneously, and turn your entire body 90° to the right.

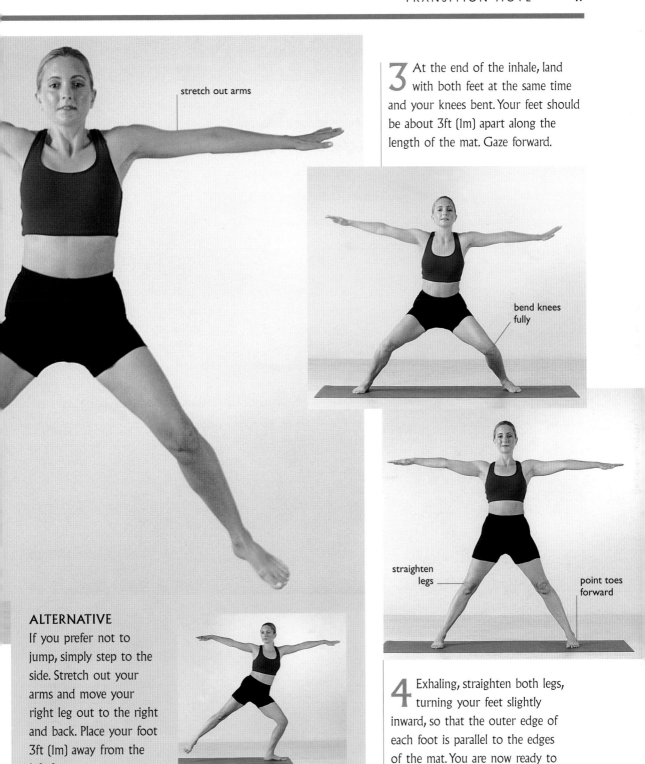

stretch out arms

3 At the end of the inhale, land with both feet at the same time and your knees bent. Your feet should be about 3ft (1m) apart along the length of the mat. Gaze forward.

bend knees fully

straighten legs

point toes forward

4 Exhaling, straighten both legs, turning your feet slightly inward, so that the outer edge of each foot is parallel to the edges of the mat. You are now ready to move into the next pose.

ALTERNATIVE
If you prefer not to jump, simply step to the side. Stretch out your arms and move your right leg out to the right and back. Place your foot 3ft (1m) away from the left foot.

UTTHITA TRIKONASANA
Extended Triangle

The extended triangle posture creates balance, poise, and sharp focus. In the Dynamic series, it is the beginning of the extended hip openers. As you practice, work with the *bandhas* to deepen the breath and improve your balance. Hold the full pose for five to eight breaths, then repeat on the left side.

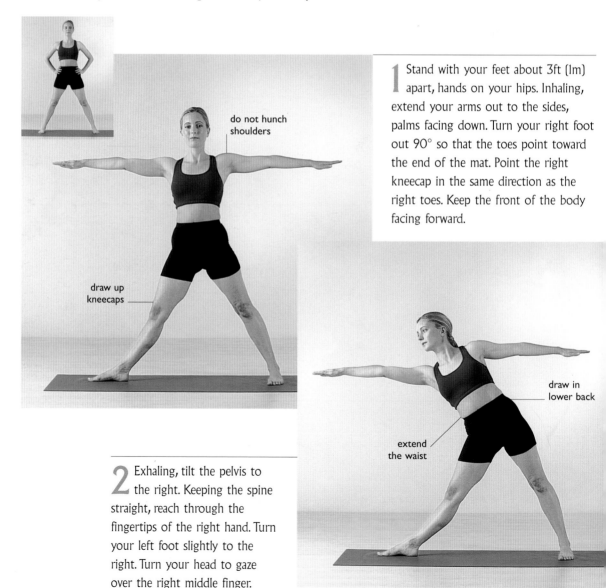

do not hunch shoulders

draw up kneecaps

draw in lower back

extend the waist

1 Stand with your feet about 3ft (1m) apart, hands on your hips. Inhaling, extend your arms out to the sides, palms facing down. Turn your right foot out 90° so that the toes point toward the end of the mat. Point the right kneecap in the same direction as the right toes. Keep the front of the body facing forward.

2 Exhaling, tilt the pelvis to the right. Keeping the spine straight, reach through the fingertips of the right hand. Turn your left foot slightly to the right. Turn your head to gaze over the right middle finger.

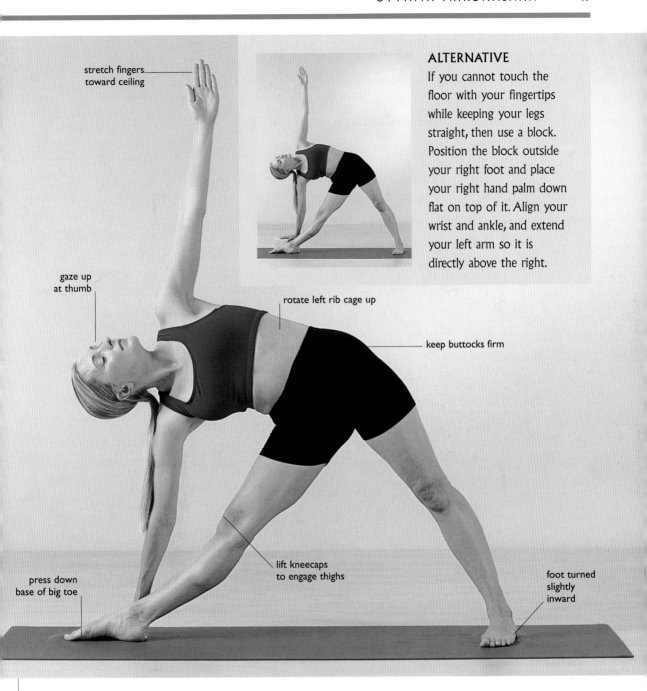

stretch fingers
toward ceiling

gaze up
at thumb

rotate left rib cage up

keep buttocks firm

lift kneecaps
to engage thighs

press down
base of big toe

foot turned
slightly
inward

ALTERNATIVE

If you cannot touch the floor with your fingertips while keeping your legs straight, then use a block. Position the block outside your right foot and place your right hand palm down flat on top of it. Align your wrist and ankle, and extend your left arm so it is directly above the right.

3 At the end of the exhale, bring the right arm down until the fingertips rest on the floor just outside the right foot. Reach up with the left arm, lengthening both sides of the torso and extending through the crown of the head. Keep both feet evenly grounded, and spread the toes. Hold the full pose for five to eight breaths. Inhale to return to step 1 and repeat on the other side. Then jump back to the top of the mat and prepare to jump out to the side (*pp.46–47*) ready for the next pose.

VIRABHADRASANA B
Warrior B

This posture forms part of the sequence of Warrior poses (*see also pp.58–59* and *74–75*). These poses are named after Virabhadra, a legendary Hindu warrior. Practicing this particular variation helps to develop strength and endurance, alleviates stiffness in the neck and shoulders, and helps to improve flexibility in the knee and hip joints. Hold the pose for five to eight breaths, then repeat on the other side.

1 With your feet wide apart, place your hands on your hips. Inhaling, turn the right foot out 90° and turn the left foot slightly inward. Extend the arms out with the palms facing downward. Turn your head to gaze at the middle finger on your right hand.

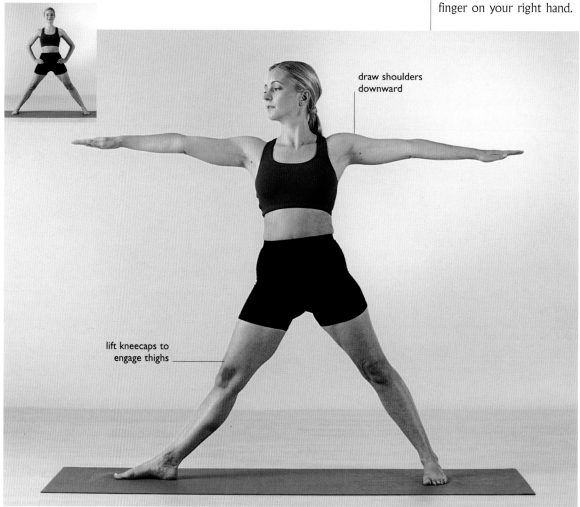

draw shoulders downward

lift kneecaps to engage thighs

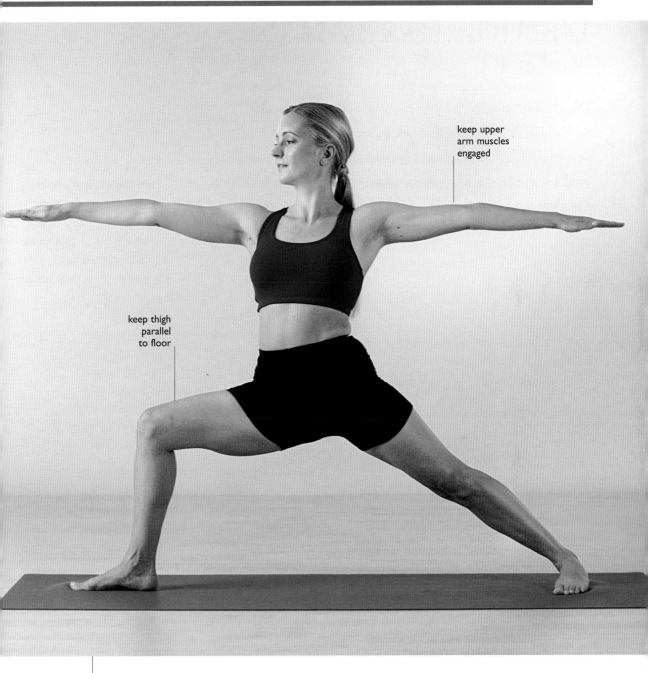

keep upper
arm muscles
engaged

keep thigh
parallel
to floor

2 Exhaling, bend your right knee so that it is over the right ankle and forms a 90° angle with your right thigh. Draw down the torso, while lifting the perineum to engage *mula bandha.* Press down the outer edge of your left foot and maintain a healthy arch. Hold the full pose for five to eight breaths. Inhale to return to step 1, and repeat on the other side. Then, jump back to the top of the mat and prepare to jump out to the side (*pp.46–47*) ready to flow into the next pose in your program.

UTTHITA PARSVAKONASANA
Extended Side Angle

This is a good pose to practice both *mula* and *uddiyana bandha*: toward the end of the exhale, contract the perineum and draw your navel to the spine. *Utthita parsvakonsanana* also releases the neck and shoulders, and trims the waist. Hold the full pose for five to eight breaths, then repeat on the left side.

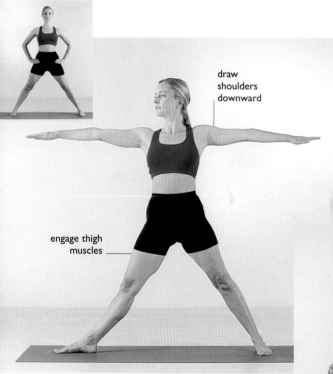

draw shoulders downward

engage thigh muscles

1 With the feet wide apart and the toes pointing forward, place your hands on your hips. Inhaling, turn the right foot out 90° and turn the left foot slightly inward. Extend the arms out to the sides and parallel to the floor with the palms facing downward. Gaze at your right middle finger.

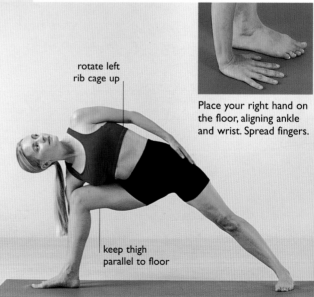

rotate left rib cage up

Place your right hand on the floor, aligning ankle and wrist. Spread fingers.

keep thigh parallel to floor

2 Exhaling, bend your right knee so it is directly over the right ankle and forms a 90° angle with the right thigh. Place your right hand, palm down, on the floor to the outside of your right foot. Rest your left hand on your hip. Gaze at the ceiling.

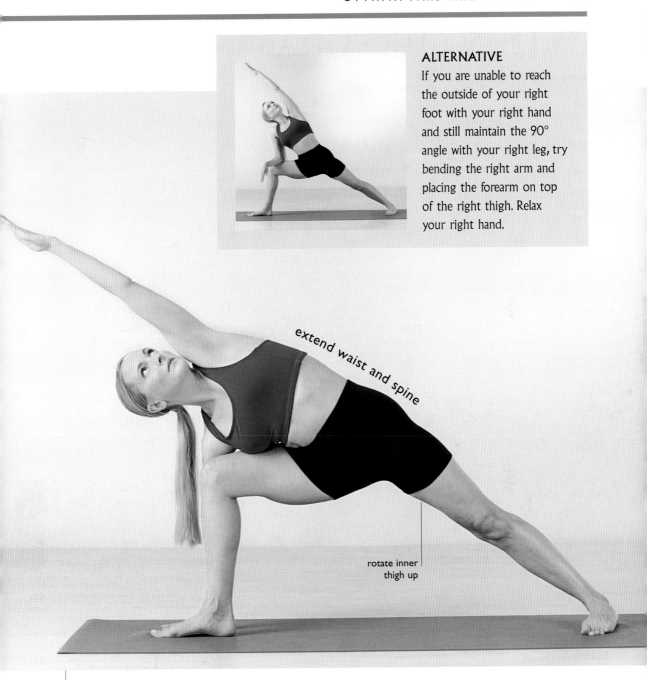

ALTERNATIVE

If you are unable to reach the outside of your right foot with your right hand and still maintain the 90° angle with your right leg, try bending the right arm and placing the forearm on top of the right thigh. Relax your right hand.

extend waist and spine

rotate inner thigh up

3 Continue exhaling as you extend your left arm over the left ear into the full pose. Stretch out through your fingertips to elongate the arm and create a straight line from the outer edge of the left foot through to the fingers. Firm the buttocks to draw in the sacrum. Turn your head toward your armpit and gaze at the center of your left palm. Hold the pose for five to eight breaths. Inhale to return to step 1, and repeat on the other side. Then jump back to the top of the mat and prepare to jump out to the side (*pp.46–47*) ready for the next pose.

ARDHA CHANDRASANA
Half Moon

The shape of the body in this pose resembles the outline of a half moon, and in Sanskrit *ardha* means "half" and *chandra* means "moon." This *asana* is excellent for improving your balance and concentration, and it also tones the lower back muscles. If you find it difficult to balance, place your back against a wall for stability. Hold the pose for five to eight breaths on the right side of the body, then repeat on the left.

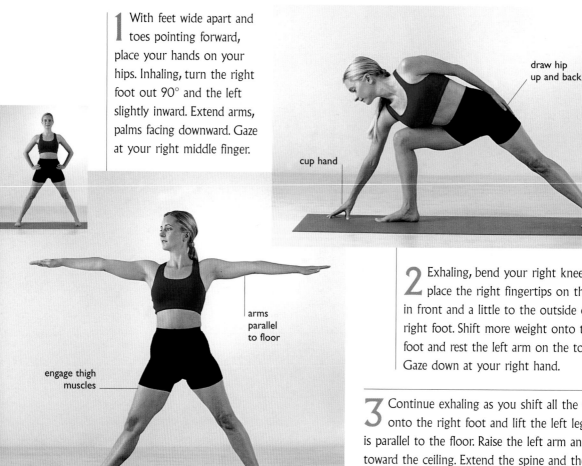

1 With feet wide apart and toes pointing forward, place your hands on your hips. Inhaling, turn the right foot out 90° and the left slightly inward. Extend arms, palms facing downward. Gaze at your right middle finger.

draw hip up and back

cup hand

arms parallel to floor

engage thigh muscles

2 Exhaling, bend your right knee and place the right fingertips on the floor in front and a little to the outside of the right foot. Shift more weight onto the right foot and rest the left arm on the torso. Gaze down at your right hand.

3 Continue exhaling as you shift all the weight onto the right foot and lift the left leg until it is parallel to the floor. Raise the left arm and point toward the ceiling. Extend the spine and the back of the neck. Hold for five to eight breaths. Inhale to return to step 1, and repeat on the other side. Jump out to the side (*pp.46–47*) ready for the next pose.

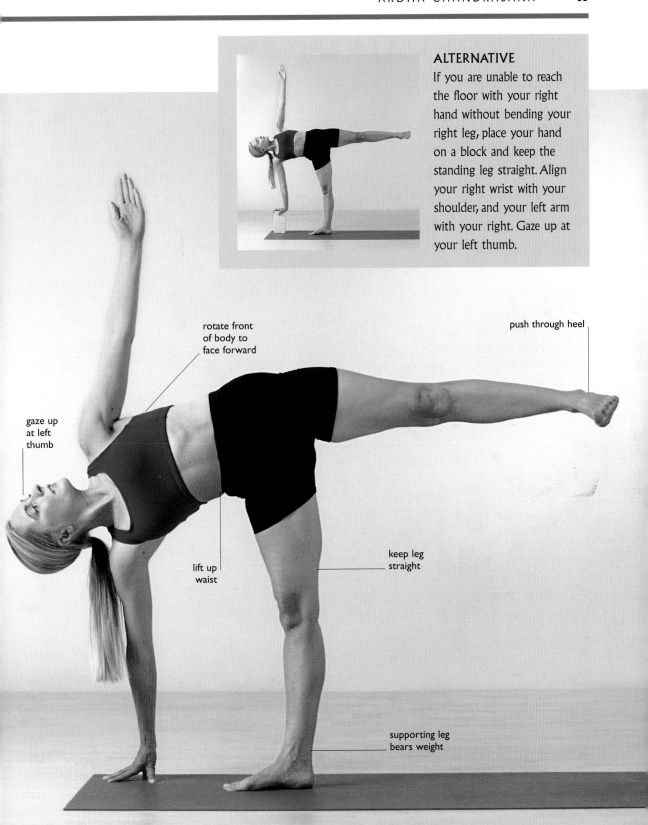

ALTERNATIVE
If you are unable to reach the floor with your right hand without bending your right leg, place your hand on a block and keep the standing leg straight. Align your right wrist with your shoulder, and your left arm with your right. Gaze up at your left thumb.

rotate front of body to face forward

push through heel

gaze up at left thumb

lift up waist

keep leg straight

supporting leg bears weight

PARSVOTTANASANA
Forward Bend to Side

In Sanskrit *parsva* means "to the side," while *uttana* means "intense stretch." The pressure of your hands on the back while they are in the reverse prayer position helps straighten the spine. The pose also releases tension in the shoulders and opens up the chest, allowing you to stretch deeply over the forward leg. This, in turn, stretches the hamstring of the forward leg. Hold the pose for five to eight breaths, then repeat on the left side of the body.

1 With feet wide apart and toes pointing forward, place your hands on your hips. Inhaling, turn the right foot and the pelvis to face the end of the mat. The left foot will turn in to accommodate the pelvic rotation.

2 Exhaling, place the hands together in the inverted prayer position, resting the little fingers on the spine. Keep the shoulders drawn down the back.

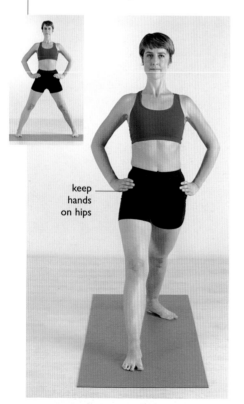

keep hands on hips

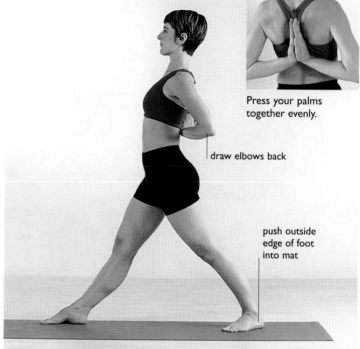

Press your palms together evenly.

draw elbows back

push outside edge of foot into mat

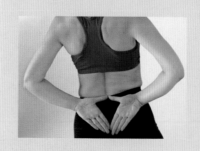

ALTERNATIVE
If you find it difficult to bring the palms of your hands together behind your back, place the backs of your hands on your lower back.

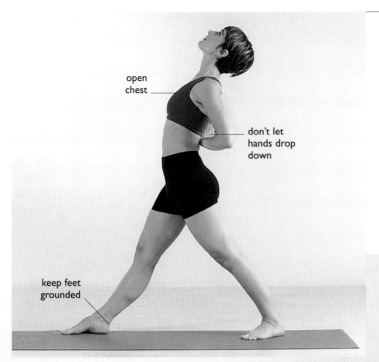

open chest

don't let hands drop down

keep feet grounded

3 Inhaling, lift up the sternum, stretch both sides of your body, and slightly arch the lower back. Gaze toward the ceiling. Do not overarch the back.

4 Exhaling, fold forward over your right leg into the full pose. Gaze toward the big toe. Hold for five to eight breaths. Inhale to return to step 1, and repeat on the other side. Then jump back to the top of the mat and out to the side (*pp.46–47*) for the next pose.

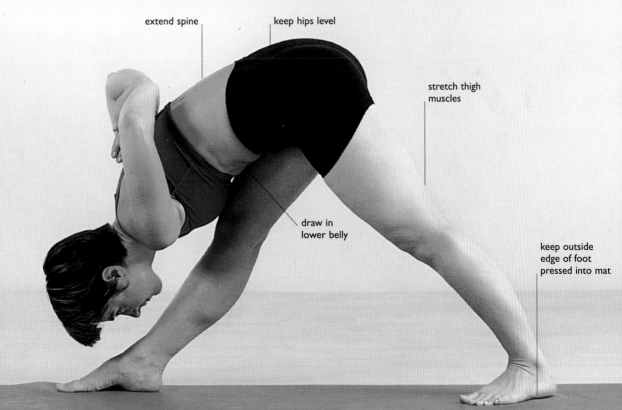

extend spine

keep hips level

stretch thigh muscles

draw in lower belly

keep outside edge of foot pressed into mat

VIRABHADRASANA A
Warrior A

In this part of the Warrior sequence, the arms are held straight up, like a warrior's sword, in the prayer position. Take on the spirit of the warrior and make your body so strong that no one can push you over. This posture helps to loosen any stiffness in the neck and reduces fat around the hips. Hold the pose for five to eight breaths, then repeat on the left.

1 With feet very wide apart and toes pointing forward, place your hands on your hips. Inhaling, turn the entire body 90° to the right. Turn the left foot inward to allow the left hip to move forward and the right hip to move back.

2 Continue inhaling as you reach out with your arms to the sides and then up to the ceiling. Place the palms of your hands together above your head in the prayer position. Gaze forward.

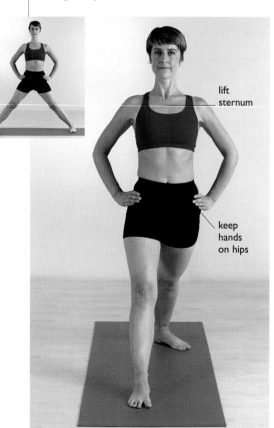

lift
sternum

keep
hands
on hips

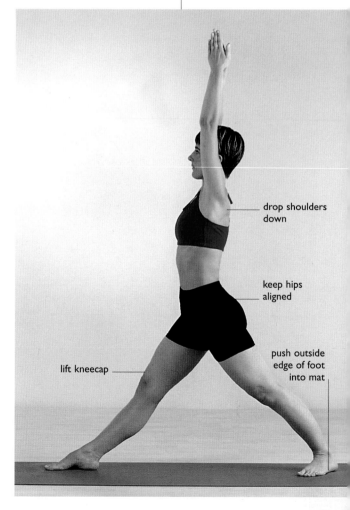

drop shoulders
down

keep hips
aligned

lift kneecap

push outside
edge of foot
into mat

3 Exhaling, bend your right knee 90° so that it is positioned above the center of your right ankle. Draw down the back of your body while lifting the perineum to engage *mula bandha.* Push the outside of the left heel and the base of the big right toe into the mat. Gaze up at your thumbs. Hold the full pose for five to eight breaths. Inhale to return to step 1, and repeat on the other side. Then jump back to the top of the mat and prepare to jump out to the side (*pp.46–47*) ready to flow into the next pose.

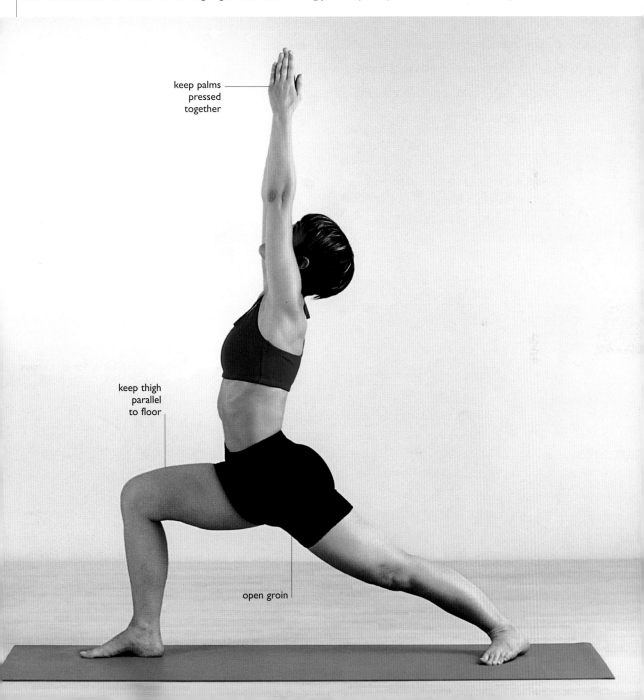

keep palms pressed together

keep thigh parallel to floor

open groin

PARIVRTTA PARSVAKONASANA
Revolving Side Angle

This pose is the counterpose to the extended side angle (*see pp. 52–53*). In this posture the spine is rotated and the abdominal muscles massaged, which aids digestion and rejuvenates the internal organs. Hold the pose for five to eight breaths, then repeat on the other side of your body.

1 With feet wide apart and toes pointing forward, place your hands on your hips. Inhaling, turn the entire body 90° to the right. Turn the left foot inward slightly to allow the left hip to move forward and the right hip to move back. Gaze forward.

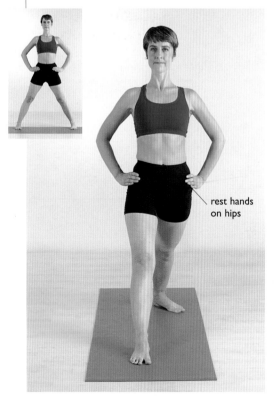

rest hands on hips

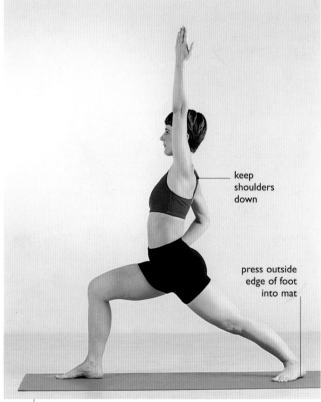

keep shoulders down

press outside edge of foot into mat

2 Continue inhaling as you bend your right knee to 90° so that it is positioned above the center of your right ankle. Keep the right thigh parallel to the floor. Reach up with your left arm and extend the spine, preparing to twist to the right. Gaze forward.

3 Exhaling, twist your torso to the right, placing the back of your left arm against the outside of your right knee. Press the outside edge of your left foot into the mat.

4 At the end of the exhale, place your left palm on the mat at the outside of the right foot. Extend the right arm over the right ear into the full pose. Gaze slightly upward. Hold for five to eight breaths. Inhale to return to step 1, and repeat on the other side. Then jump back to the top of the mat and out to the side (*pp.46–47*) for the next pose.

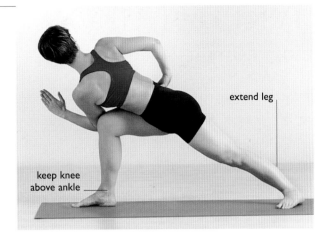

extend leg

keep knee above ankle

ALTERNATIVE

If your hand cannot reach the ground, place your left arm on top of the right thigh and put the hands together in the prayer position. Keep reaching up with your right elbow.

Place the left hand flat outside the right foot.

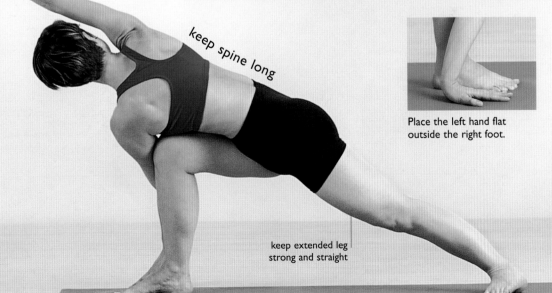

keep spine long

keep extended leg strong and straight

PARIVRTTA TRIKONASANA
Revolving Triangle

This *asana* is the counterpose to the extended triangle (*pp.48–49*). In addition to toning the thighs and calf muscles, this pose can relieve back tension because, as with all revolving poses, the abdominal organs are rejuvenated and the hip muscles stretched. Remember to engage *mula bandha* to help you balance, and use a block if you need to. Hold the full pose for five to eight breaths, then repeat on the left side of the body.

1 With feet wide apart and toes pointing forward, place your hands on your hips. Inhaling, turn your entire body 90° to the right. Turn your left foot slightly inward.

2 Continue inhaling and reach up with your left arm and extend the spine. Pull the right hip back and move the left hip forward.

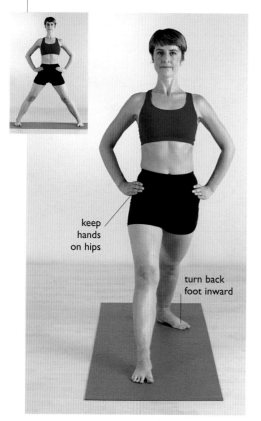

keep hands on hips

turn back foot inward

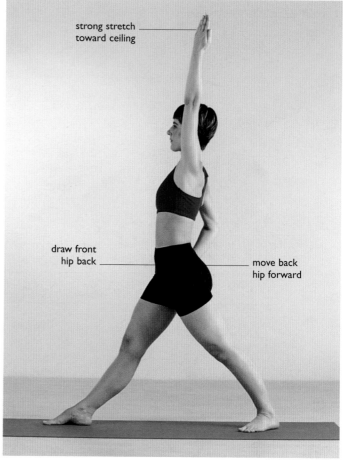

strong stretch toward ceiling

draw front hip back

move back hip forward

3 Exhaling, bend your torso sideways to the left and place your left palm to the outside of your right foot. Keep the shoulder blades pushed down the back.

4 At the end of the exhale, reach straight up with the fingertips of your right hand. Revolve your torso out from your hips. Inhale to return to step 1, and repeat on the other side. Jump back to the top of the mat and out to the side (*pp.46–47*) for the next pose.

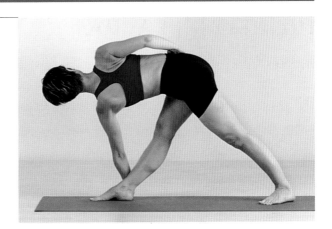

ALTERNATIVE
If you cannot reach the floor with your left hand without bending your right leg, place your left hand, palm down, on a block positioned just to the outside of your right foot. Align your wrist with your ankle.

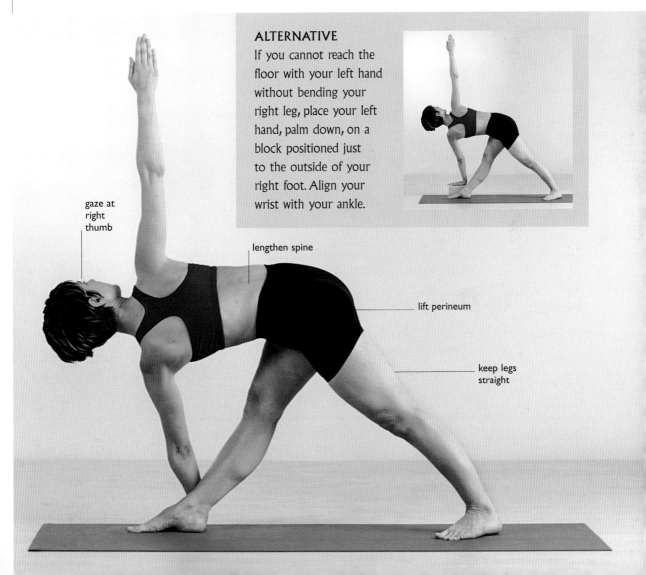

gaze at
right
thumb

lengthen spine

lift perineum

keep legs
straight

PRASARITA PADOTTANASANA A
Foot Spreading A

This pose is particularly useful for those unable to do headstands. Do not worry if you cannot reach the floor with the crown of your head: this will come with practice. This posture expands and stretches the legs, develops the hamstrings and adductor muscles, as well as improving digestion. Hold the full pose for five to eight breaths.

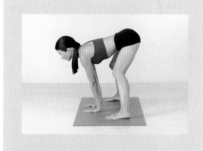

ALTERNATIVE
If you cannot reach the floor with your hands while keeping your legs straight, bend your knees until your hands are flat on the floor. Gaze forward.

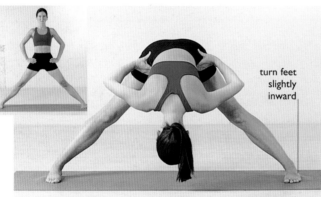

turn feet slightly inward

1 With your feet wide apart and your toes pointing forward, place your hands on your hips. Exhaling, fold your body forward. Keep your shoulders wide and pulled toward the hips. Gaze back between your legs.

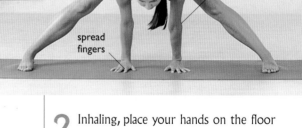

straighten arms

spread fingers

2 Inhaling, place your hands on the floor shoulder-width apart between your feet. Lift the torso. Lengthen the spine and the back of your neck. Gaze forward and slightly upward.

whole sequence at a glance

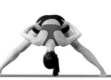
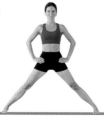
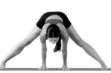

Inhaling.....................Exhaling.............................Inhaling................

3 Exhaling, bend the elbows to lower the crown of your head to the floor between your hands. Do not force your head to the floor as this will curve the spine. Extend your spine and lower your head as far as you can. Lift your shoulders away from the floor. Gaze back between the legs. Hold the full pose for five to eight breaths.

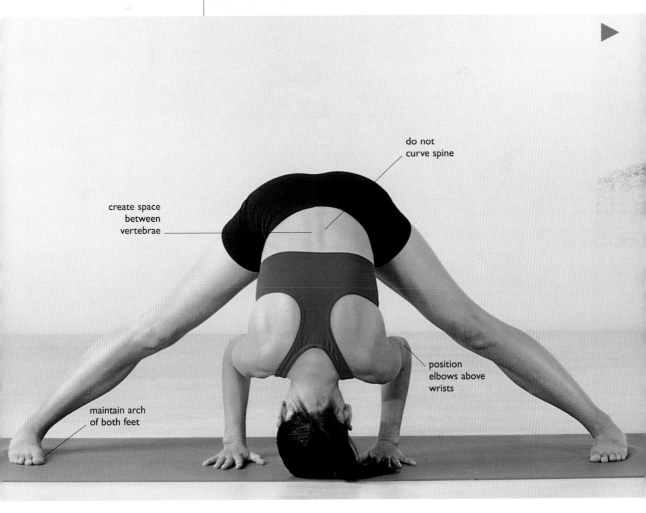

do not
curve spine

create space
between
vertebrae

position
elbows above
wrists

maintain arch
of both feet

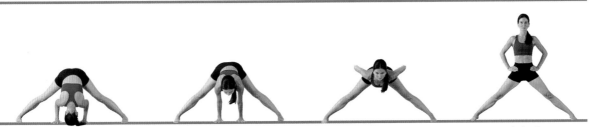

..........Exhaling..................Inhaling..................Exhaling..................Inhaling.......

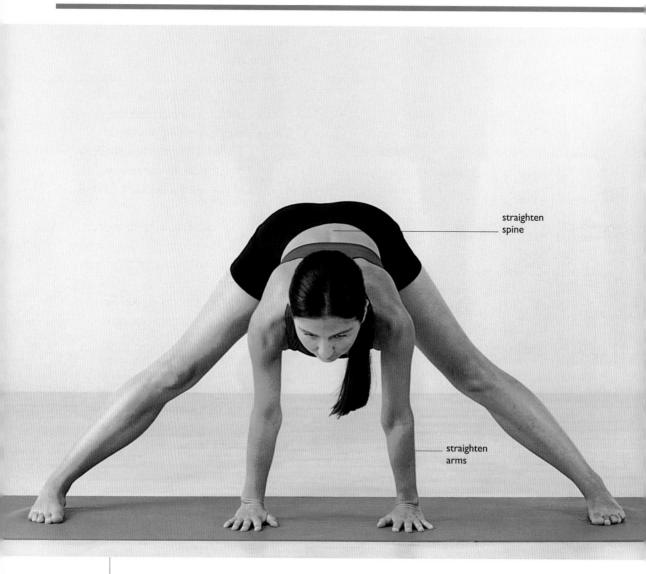

straighten
spine

straighten
arms

4 Inhaling, straighten your arms, while
keeping your hands flat on the floor.
Lift up the torso to straighten the spine,
taking care not to overarch the back.
Gaze forward and slightly upward.

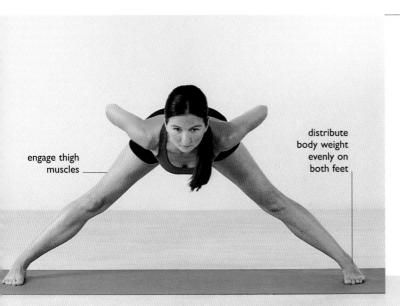

engage thigh
muscles

distribute
body weight
evenly on
both feet

5 Exhaling, place your hands on your hips with the thumbs pointing toward the buttocks. Keeping the spine long and straight, lift the sternum, preparing to stand. Gaze forward.

6 Inhaling, bring your body up to standing keeping your hands on your hips. Next, jump back to the top of the mat and out to the side (*pp.46–47*) ready to flow into the next pose.

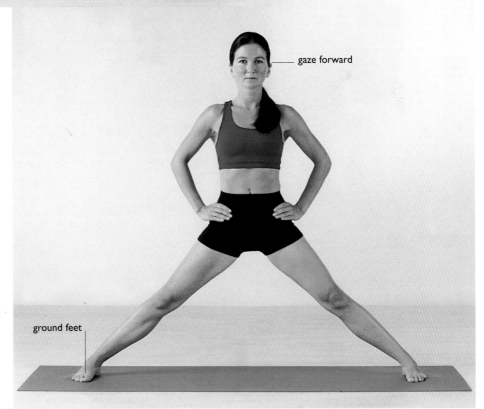

gaze forward

ground feet

PADANGUSTHASANA & PADAHASTASANA
Big Toe, & Hand & Foot Forward Bend

These postures are standing forward bends that improve the functioning and control of the perineal muscles used when engaging *mula bandha*. If you suffer from lower back tension, it is important to bend the knees and keep the spine stable. Hold both the full poses for five to eight breaths.

2 Still exhaling, grab hold of both big toes. Reach toward the floor with the crown of your head. Gaze back between your legs and engage *mula bandha*. Hold *Padangusthasana* for five to eight breaths.

1 Stand with your feet hip-width apart and your hands on your hips. Exhaling, fold your body forward, keeping the spine straight.

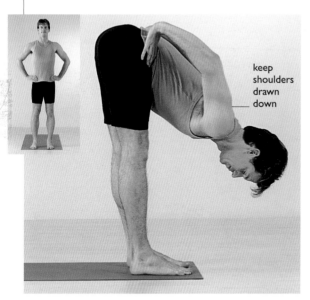

keep shoulders drawn down

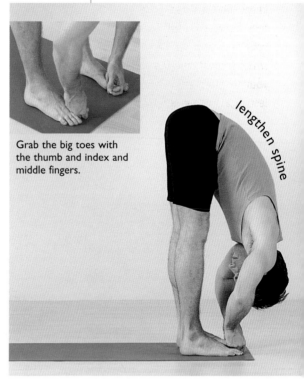

Grab the big toes with the thumb and index and middle fingers.

lengthen spine

whole sequence at a glance

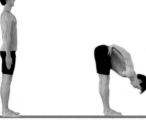

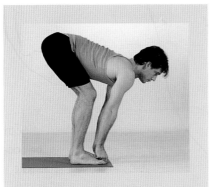

ALTERNATIVE

If you cannot reach your toes with straight legs, bend at the knees until you can grasp your toes firmly while still keeping your arms straight. Keep your wrists straight, and distribute your weight evenly over both feet. Gaze slightly forward.

3 Inhaling, lift up the torso, while holding the toes firmly and straightening the arms. Gaze slightly forward.

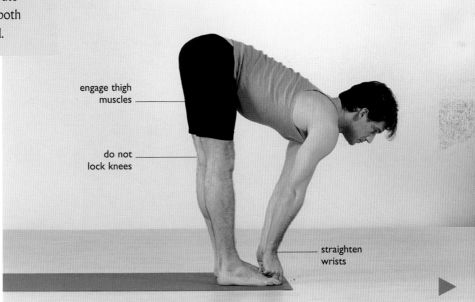

engage thigh muscles

do not lock knees

straighten wrists

  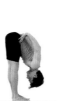 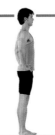 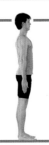

....Finish inhaling..........Begin exhaling........Finish exhaling........Inhaling..........Exhaling

4 Still inhaling, keep the torso half-way up and spread your toes. Place your hands under your feet, so that the undersides of your toes rest on the palms of your hands and the tops of your hands are on the floor. Gaze slightly forward.

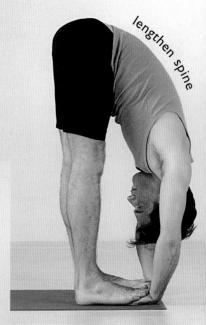

lengthen spine

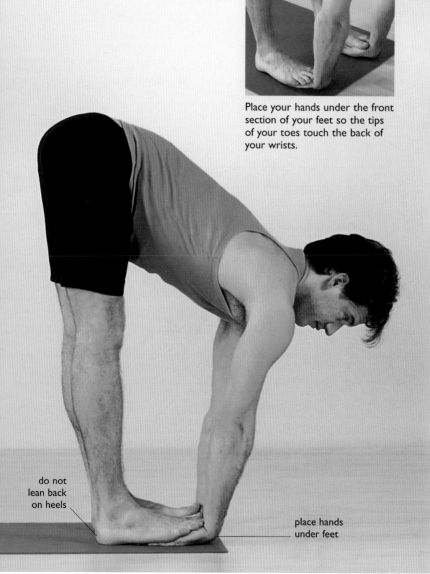

Place your hands under the front section of your feet so the tips of your toes touch the back of your wrists.

5 Exhaling, fold forward again, extending the crown of the head toward the floor. Bend your arms slightly, so that your elbows point out to the sides. Draw the shoulders down the back and gaze at the navel. Engage *mula bandha*. Hold *Padahastasana* for five to eight breaths.

do not lean back on heels

place hands under feet

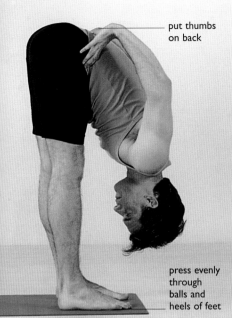

put thumbs on back

press evenly through balls and heels of feet

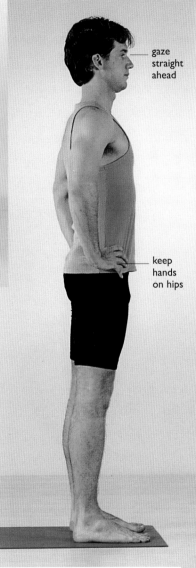

gaze straight ahead

keep hands on hips

6 Exhaling, bring your arms up to place your hands on your hips. Keep your weight forward in the feet and press down with the heels.

7 Inhaling, lift the torso back to standing, while keeping your hands on your hips. Keep your legs straight and gaze straight ahead.

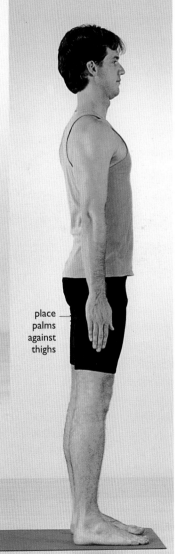

place palms against thighs

8 Exhaling, stand straight and tall with your arms down by the sides of your torso. Gaze forward. Stay in this position for the next pose.

VRKSASANA
Tree

In Sanskrit *vrksa* means "tree," and this posture creates a strong, rooted stance, just as a tree's roots grow deeper into the earth and its branches reach up to the sky, stabilizing the tree. The pose strengthens the leg muscles and develops balance. Lift the perineum throughout to improve balance. Hold the pose for five to eight breaths on the left leg, then repeat on the right. If you are combining this pose with Warrior C (*see pp.74–75*), complete both poses on the left before switching to the right.

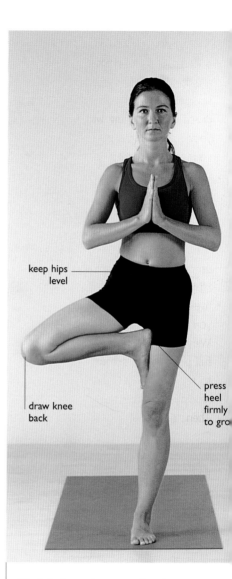

keep hips level

draw knee back

press heel firmly to gro

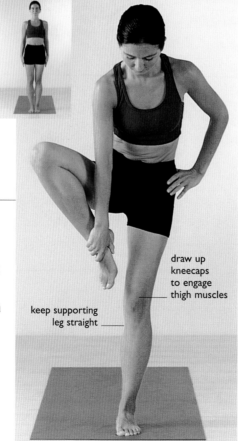

draw up kneecaps to engage thigh muscles

keep supporting leg straight

1 With your feet together and arms by your side, inhale as you reach forward and grab your right ankle. Place the right foot on the inner left thigh. Keep the right heel as close to the groin as possible, with the toes pointing down.

2 Exhaling, place your hands together in the prayer postion. Lift the sternum and stand up very straight. Do not let the shoulders hunch. Gaze forward. Hold your gaze soft and steady to help you balance.

3 Inhaling, extend the arms up and press the palms together while straightening the arms. Reach for the ceiling with your fingertips and root your left heel to the floor to lengthen the spine. Keep your right foot pressed firmly into the groin to prevent it from sliding. Gaze upward at your thumbs. Hold the full pose for five to eight breaths. If you are also practicing Warrior C, remain in the full pose. If not, exhale to return to step 1, and repeat on the left side. Then stand with your feet together and arms by your sides ready to flow into the next pose.

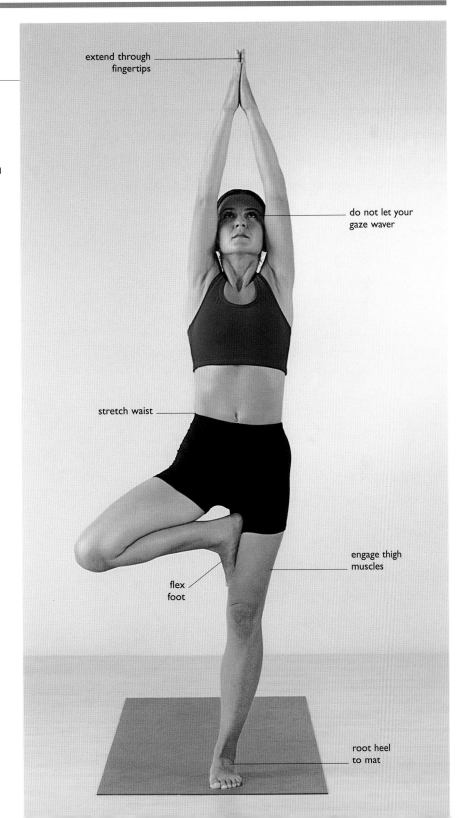

extend through fingertips

do not let your gaze waver

stretch waist

engage thigh muscles

flex foot

root heel to mat

VIRABHADRASANA C
Warrior C

Like the Tree pose on pages 72–73, Warrior C strengthens the leg muscles and improves your sense of balance, encouraging a graceful stance. To help you maintain your balance in the full pose, engage *uddiyana bandha* by drawing your navel to the spine. Hold the full pose for five to eight breaths, then return to step 1 of *Vrksasana* (pp.72–73) and repeat on the other side.

1 Starting from the Tree pose (*p.73*), exhale and start to stretch your right leg back and the torso forward. Keep your left leg straight and the arms stretched out in front, the palms together, as you prepare to extend the body until it is parallel to the floor. Gaze down slightly, and hold your gaze soft and steady to help keep your balance.

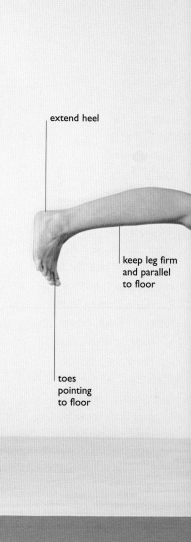

extend heel

keep leg firm and parallel to floor

toes pointing to floor

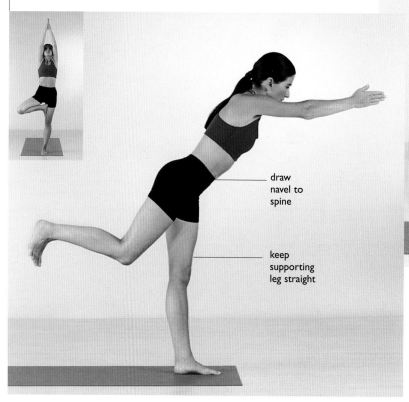

draw navel to spine

keep supporting leg straight

2 At the end of the exhale, extend your right leg fully. Turn the right kneecap and toes to face down. Gaze at the floor between your arms. Hold the full pose for five to eight breaths.

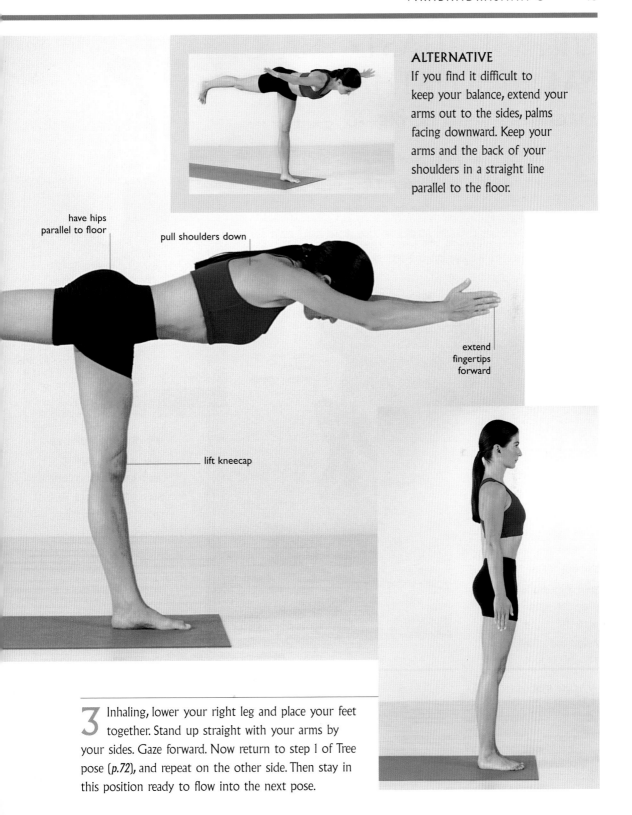

ALTERNATIVE

If you find it difficult to keep your balance, extend your arms out to the sides, palms facing downward. Keep your arms and the back of your shoulders in a straight line parallel to the floor.

have hips parallel to floor

pull shoulders down

extend fingertips forward

lift kneecap

3 Inhaling, lower your right leg and place your feet together. Stand up straight with your arms by your sides. Gaze forward. Now return to step 1 of Tree pose (*p.72*), and repeat on the other side. Then stay in this position ready to flow into the next pose.

UTTHITA HASTA PADANGUSTHASANA
Extended Hand & Big Toe

You need to engage both *mula bandha* and *uddiyana bandha* throughout to maintain the balance and form of this posture, which benefits the kidneys, perineum, and the abdominal and leg muscles. There are two key stages to this pose: hold each for five to eight breaths. Repeat on the left side of the body.

lift sternum

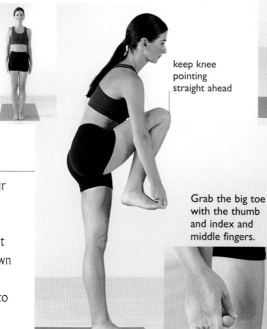

keep knee pointing straight ahead

1 Stand tall with your feet together and arms by your sides. Exhaling, lift your right knee up and reach down the outside of the leg with your right hand to grab the right big toe with the thumb and index and middle fingers.

Grab the big toe with the thumb and index and middle fingers.

2 Inhaling, stand up straight, pulling your knee to the chest. Keep your left leg very straight and firm. Gaze straight ahead.

whole sequence at a glance

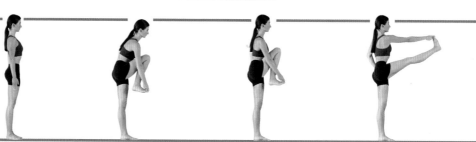

Inhaling..............Exhaling................Inhaling..........Exhaling, then inhaling.....

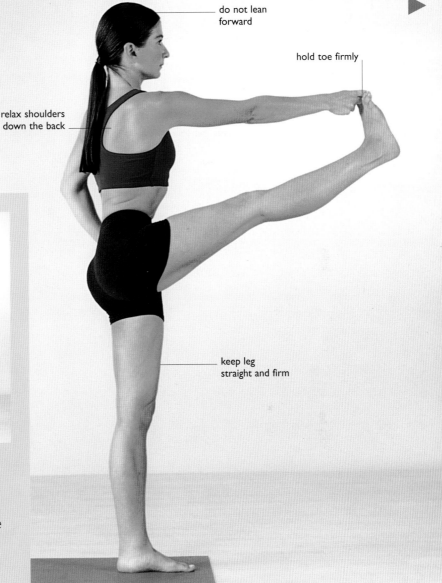

3 Exhaling, extend your right leg as straight as possible into the first of the full-pose stages. Extend your right heel and the base of the big toe while standing up straight. Use a strap if necessary. Hold for five to eight breaths.

do not lean forward

hold toe firmly

relax shoulders down the back

keep leg straight and firm

ALTERNATIVE

If you cannot extend your leg out straight in front of you, keep the leg bent and hold the front of the knee with your hand. Pull the knee close to the chest, standing very tall.

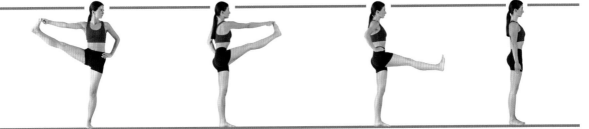

. . . . Exhaling . . . . Inhaling . . . . Exhaling, then inhaling . . . . Exhaling . . . .

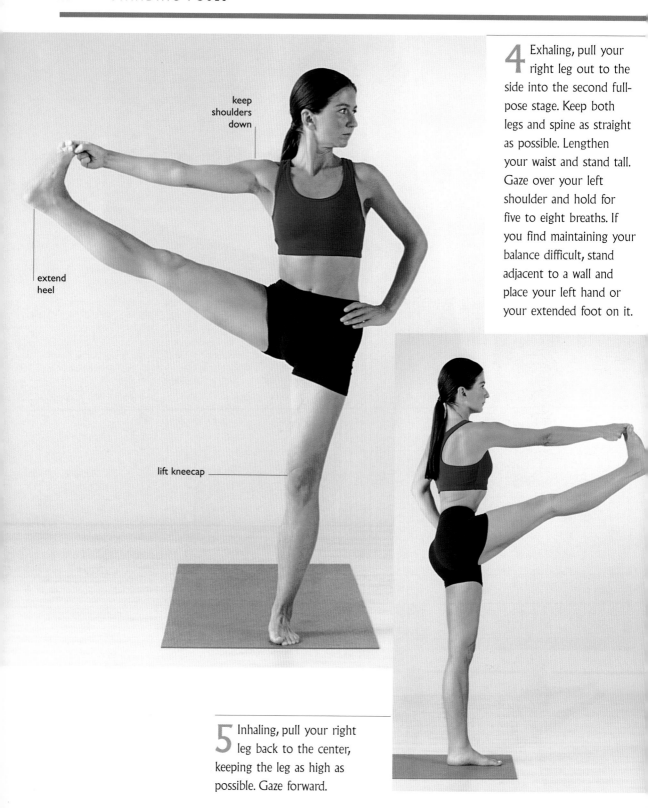

keep
shoulders
down

extend
heel

lift kneecap

4 Exhaling, pull your right leg out to the side into the second full-pose stage. Keep both legs and spine as straight as possible. Lengthen your waist and stand tall. Gaze over your left shoulder and hold for five to eight breaths. If you find maintaining your balance difficult, stand adjacent to a wall and place your left hand or your extended foot on it.

5 Inhaling, pull your right leg back to the center, keeping the leg as high as possible. Gaze forward.

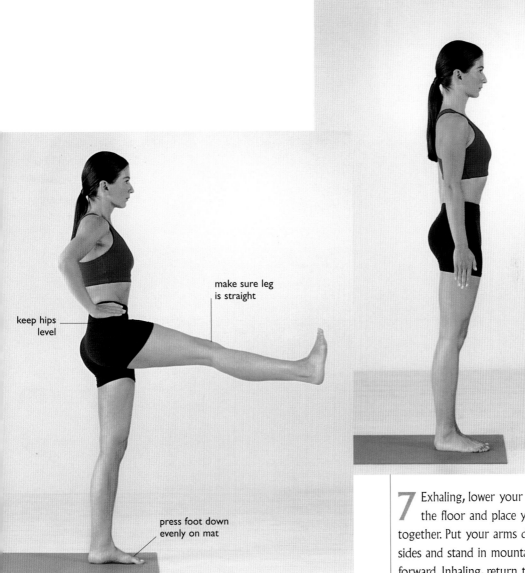

keep hips
level

make sure leg
is straight

press foot down
evenly on mat

6 Exhaling, release your right foot and rest your hands on your waist. Let the leg float. Keep your chest open and lifted. Relax the face. Gaze forward. Hold this pose for one complete inhalation.

7 Exhaling, lower your right leg to the floor and place your feet together. Put your arms down by your sides and stand in mountain pose. Gaze forward. Inhaling, return to step 1, and repeat on the other side. Then stay in this position ready for the next pose.

BACKWARD BENDS

Now we move into the backward bending postures, which are more dynamic than the standing *asanas*. Backward bends can be very exhilarating, but are also challenging. Do not push your body beyond what it can comfortably achieve. Rather, bring awareness to your body's limitations, and with repeated practice gradually move deeper into each pose.

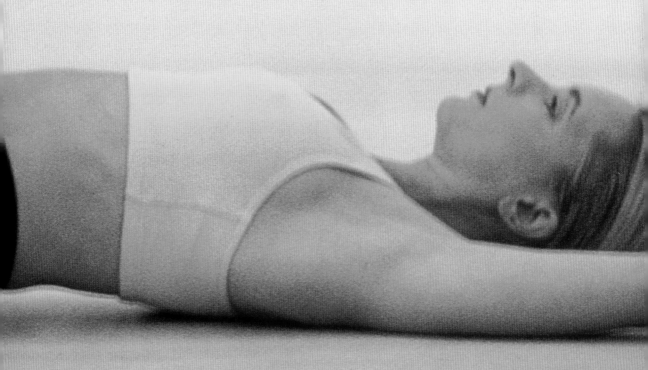

TRANSITION MOVE
Standing to Lying on Belly

The essence of dynamic yoga is the transition from one pose to another using some of the graceful steps of the Sun Salutations. This sequence takes you from your last standing position to lying on your belly in preparation for the first backward bend posture. Follow the breathing pattern closely.

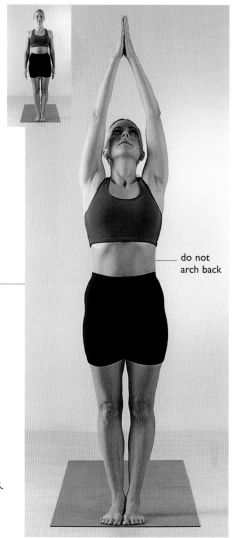

do not arch back

1 Standing tall with your feet together and arms by your sides, inhale and stretch your arms out and upward, bringing the palms together above your head. Extend through your fingertips, pushing your heels into the mat. Gaze up at your thumbs.

2 Exhaling, fold the body forward, drawing back the pubic bone and lifting up the sitting bones. Place your hands flat on the floor at the outside of your feet and parallel to them. Keep your legs straight. Relax your neck and gaze toward the front of your legs.

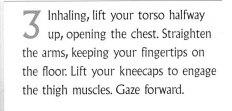

extend spine

3 Inhaling, lift your torso halfway up, opening the chest. Straighten the arms, keeping your fingertips on the floor. Lift your kneecaps to engage the thigh muscles. Gaze forward.

4 Begin exhaling and bend your knees in a crouching position. Place your palms on the floor. Keep your arms straight. Still exhaling, step back with your right foot and then the left foot. Place hip-width apart in the pre-plank position.

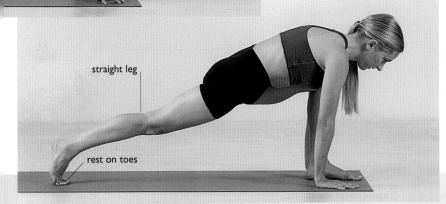

straight leg

rest on toes

5 Inhaling, keep the arms straight and look down. Draw the navel to the spine, and fully engage both the front and back of the body, preparing to flow into the next pose.

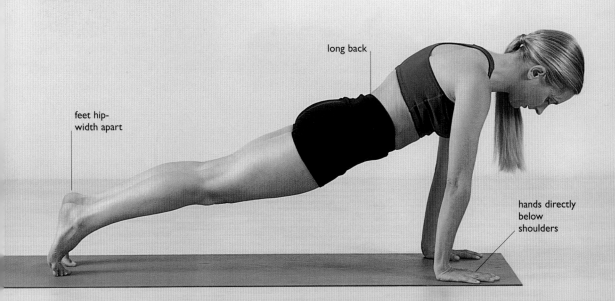

long back

feet hip-width apart

hands directly below shoulders

SALABHASANA
Locust

In Sanskrit *salabha* means "locust," and this posture resembles a locust resting on the ground. There are two key stages in this pose, both of which help to increase the flexibility of the spine and improve digestion. Hold the first stage for three to five breaths, then rest for a moment with the arms and legs on the floor. Then hold the second stage for three to five breaths. Be careful not to strain your back.

1 Exhaling, from the pre-plank position (*p.83*), fully engage the body and lower it evenly until it rests on the floor. Keep your elbows in very close to the sides of your torso and gaze down at the floor.

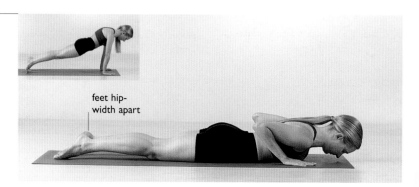

feet hip-width apart

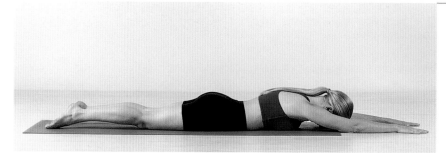

2 Continue exhaling as you extend your arms straight out above your head. Place the palms of your hands and your forehead on the floor.

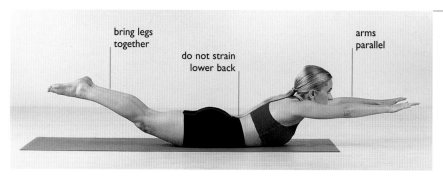

bring legs together

do not strain lower back

arms parallel

3 Inhaling, lift your arms and legs off the floor as far as you can. Keep the pubic bone and stomach on the floor. Gaze ahead. Hold this key stage of the pose for three to five breaths.

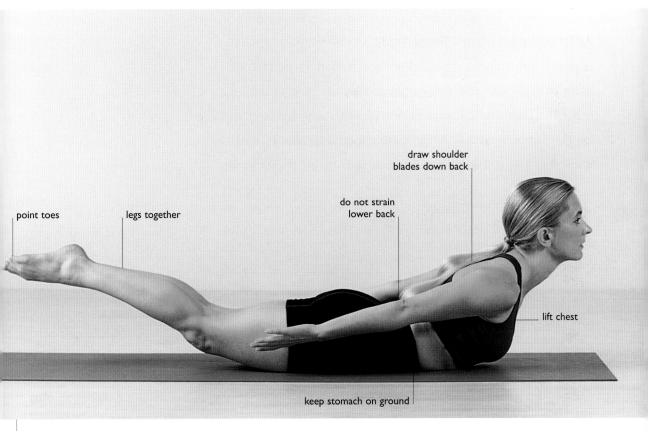

draw shoulder
blades down back

do not strain
lower back

point toes

legs together

lift chest

keep stomach on ground

4 Exhaling, lower your legs
and arms to the floor. Bring
your arms by the side of your
body, palms facing upward.
Inhaling, go into the second key
stage of this pose. Lift your arms
and legs off the floor again as far
as you can without straining the
lower back. Keep your shoulders
pulled down the back and your
chest open. Hold for three to five
breaths. Gaze forward.

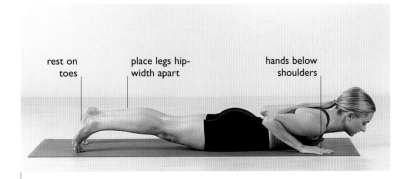

rest on
toes

place legs hip-
width apart

hands below
shoulders

5 Exhaling, lower your legs to the floor, resting on your toes. Place
your hands on the floor near your chest and elbows close to the
body. Hold your head up slightly, so your chin is just above the mat.
You are now ready to flow into the next pose.

TRANSITION MOVE
Locust to Bow

From the Locust you can if you wish go into a transitional series of poses that continues the flowing rhythm of the dynamic series. These postures are very helpful in stretching the front of the body. They also release the lower back just in case any unneccesary tension has been created during the previous back-bending postures. Make sure that you follow the specific breathing patterns described.

1 Lying on your front, with your hands just below the shoulders and feet hip-width apart, inhale and roll forward onto the tops of your feet into *Urdhva mukha svanasana (p.24)*. Lift up the chest and keep the legs firm and lifted. Gaze up.

2 Exhaling, lift your hips up and back, rolling back over your toes into *Adho mukha svanasana (p.25)*. Press your heels to the floor and push through the base of your fingers to stretch the arms. Gaze back.

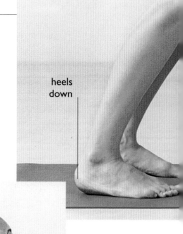

heels down

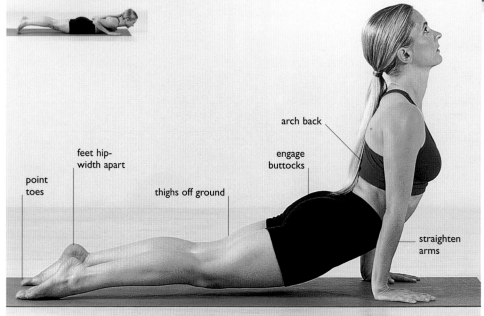

arch back

engage buttocks

feet hip-width apart

point toes

thighs off ground

straighten arms

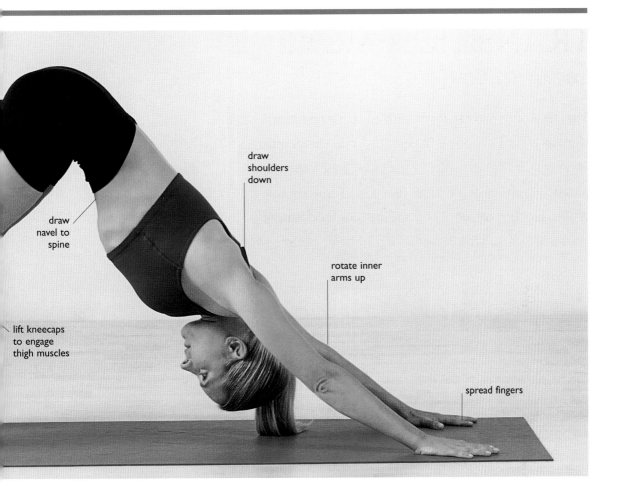

draw
shoulders
down

draw
navel to
spine

rotate inner
arms up

lift kneecaps
to engage
thigh muscles

spread fingers

3 Inhaling, shift the torso forward, bringing your legs down toward the floor. Keep the spine and legs in a straight line. Pull the navel to the spine to engage *uddiyana bandha,* and engage the buttocks. Gaze down.

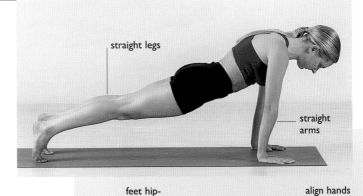

straight legs

straight
arms

feet hip-
width apart

align hands
with shoulders

4 Exhaling, lower your body to the floor, keeping your hands just below the shoulders, and elbows close to the torso. Rest your chin on the mat. Remain where you are for the next pose.

DHANURASANA
Bow

In Sanskrit *dhanu* means "bow," and in this pose, the arms are the bow-string and
the trunk and legs are arched like the bow. This posture increases the elasticity
of the spine and tones the abdominal organs. It is important not to create
tension in your lower back or strain the knees trying to reach the ankles.
If you cannot reach your ankles, lift your legs and extend your hands back
toward the feet. Hold the full pose for five breaths. Repeat the sequence twice.

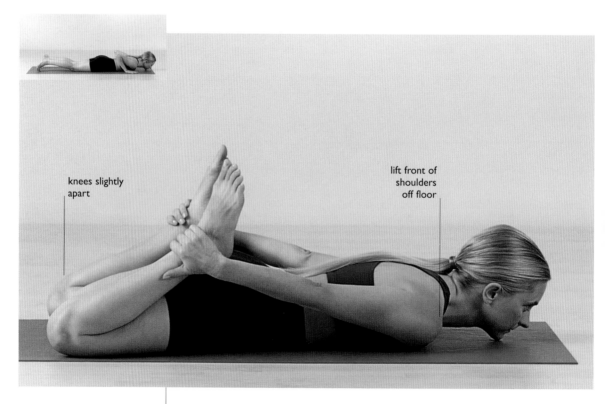

knees slightly
apart

lift front of
shoulders
off floor

1 Lying on your front, with your hands
just below the shoulders, inhale and
bend the legs back. Keep the pubic bone
pressed to the mat. Stretch the arms back
and grab hold of the ankles firmly with
both hands. Exhale completely.

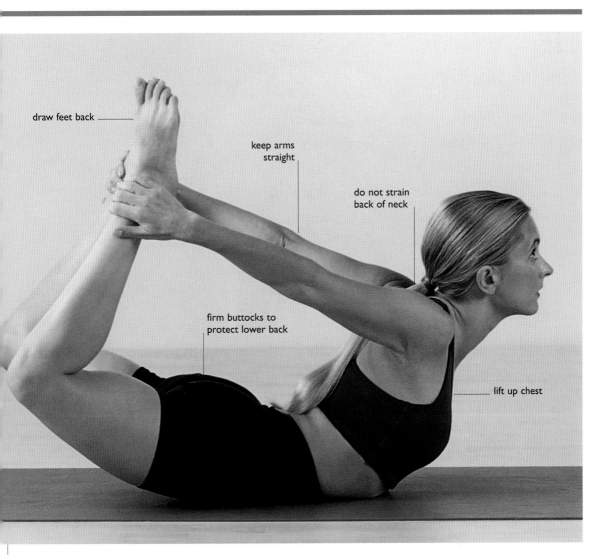

draw feet back

keep arms
straight

do not strain
back of neck

firm buttocks to
protect lower back

lift up chest

2 Inhaling, lift your legs and chest off the mat into the full pose. Pull the shins away from your hands, allowing the arms to stretch and the back to arch. Hold for five breaths.

3 Exhaling, release your ankles and lower your legs and chest. Place your hands flat on the floor and your chin on the mat. Return to step 1, and repeat the sequence. Stay in this position for the next pose.

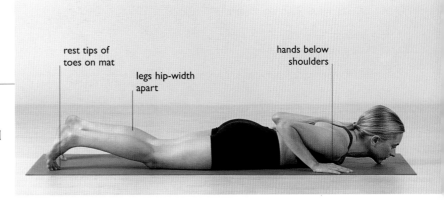

rest tips of
toes on mat

legs hip-width
apart

hands below
shoulders

TRANSITION MOVE
Bow to Sitting

This sequence shows the transition moves from lying on your stomach to sitting. Jumping to a sitting position is excellent for strengthening the abdominal muscles and learning how to lift the body effortlessly. Follow the breath pattern to learn how to synchronize the movement and breath.

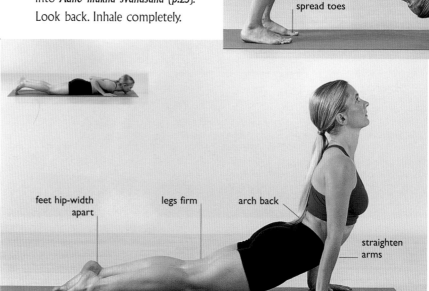

draw navel to spine

engage thigh muscles

spread toes

2 Exhaling, lift your hips up and back, pushing the sitting bones toward the ceiling into *Adho mukha svanasana* (*p.25*). Look back. Inhale completely.

1 Lying on your front, with the tips of your toes touching the floor, inhale and push your torso forward and lift your chest to move into *Urdhva mukha svanasana* (*p.24*). Balance on the tops of your feet, keeping the legs lifted off the mat. Stretch the front of the body, from the pubic bone to the sternum. Gaze up.

feet hip-width apart

legs firm

arch back

straighten arms

whole sequence at a glance

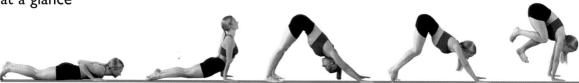

Exhaling.................Inhaling........Exhaling, then inhaling...Begin exhaling...Continue exhali

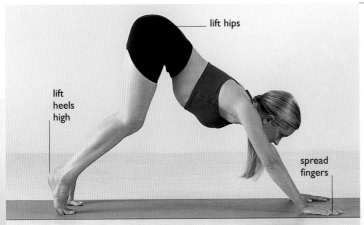

lift hips

lift
heels
high

spread
fingers

keep arms
straight

3 Begin exhaling, bend your knees, and lift your heels off the mat so you are balancing on the balls of your feet. Gaze slightly forward between your hands.

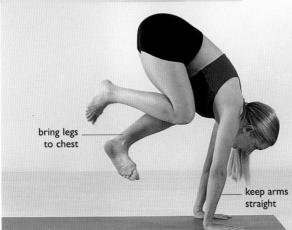

bring legs
to chest

keep arms
straight

4 Continue exhaling and, shifting your weight onto your hands, push off the feet and cross the legs in mid-air, compacting the torso. Gaze between hands.

5 At the end of the exhale, land with your feet crossed as close to your hands as possible. Remain in a squatting position.

rest on
balls
of feet

hands flat

....Finish exhaling........Begin inhaling........Finish inhaling.............Exhaling.............Inhaling

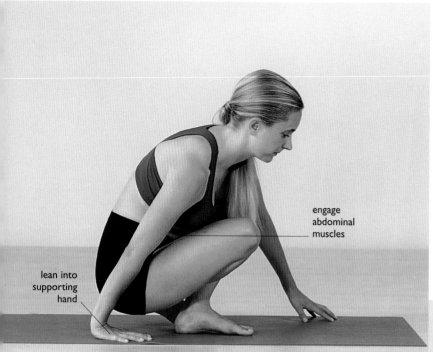

engage
abdominal
muscles

lean into
supporting
hand

6 Inhaling, place your right hand behind the right hip with the palm flat on the floor and facing forward. Lean back on the right hand, so it supports the weight of your body. Keep your left heel on the floor.

7 Continue inhaling and place your left hand behind your left hip. Lean back on both hands, keeping the buttocks off the floor by engaging the lower abdominal muscles.

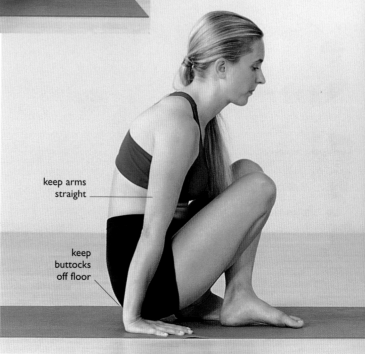

keep arms
straight

keep
buttocks
off floor

8 Begin exhaling as you extend and straighten both legs at the same time. Engage *mula bandha* and keep the buttocks off the mat until the heels touch the mat. Let your hands support your weight. Gaze forward at your big toes.

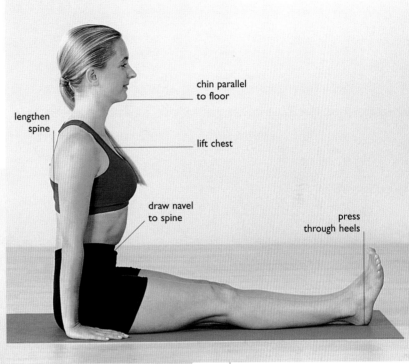

chin parallel to floor

lengthen spine

lift chest

draw navel to spine

press through heels

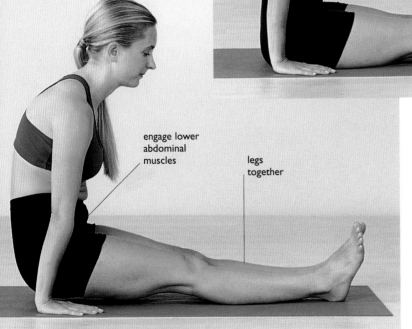

engage lower abdominal muscles

legs together

9 At the end of the exhale, rest the buttocks on the floor and sit up straight with your hands next to your hips in the seated staff pose, *Dandasana*. Press through the heels. Gaze forward. Inhale completely. You are now ready to flow into the next pose.

URDHVA DHANURASANA
Upward Bow

In Sanskrit *urdhva* means "upward" and *dhanu* means "bow."
In this posture the body is arched like a bow, which is
wonderful for releasing the entire front of the body, opening
the chest, and improving the depth of the breath. If you have
any back injuries, consult a physician before attempting the
pose or do the alternative. Hold the full pose for five breaths
and repeat two to three times.

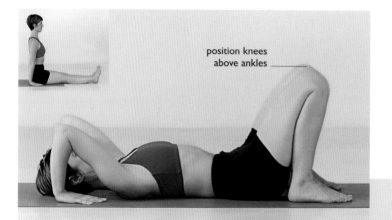

position knees
above ankles

2 Inhaling, lift up your hips and
place the crown of your head
on the floor. Push evenly through
your feet and hands. Your weight
should be distributed between
your hands and feet. Gaze forward.

1 Begin in *Dandasana,* your legs
stretched out in front of you
and your palms on the floor at
your sides. Exhaling, lie down,
bend your knees, and place your
feet flat on the floor and slightly
wider apart than the hips. Keep
the feet pointing straight
throughout the posture. Place
your hands above your shoulders,
palms flat, with your fingertips
facing the same way as your feet.

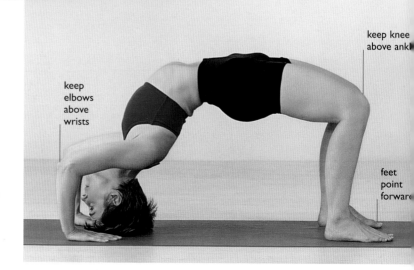

keep
elbows
above
wrists

keep knee
above ankl

feet
point
forward

3 Exhale to establish *mula bandha*. Inhaling, press through your feet and hands, lifting the hips high and straightening the arms. Lift and widen the armpits. Engage the buttocks and thighs. Gaze forward. Hold for five breaths.

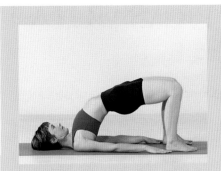

ALTERNATIVE
Press evenly through your feet and engage the thigh muscles to lift the hips as high as possible while keeping your shoulders on the floor. Gaze forward.

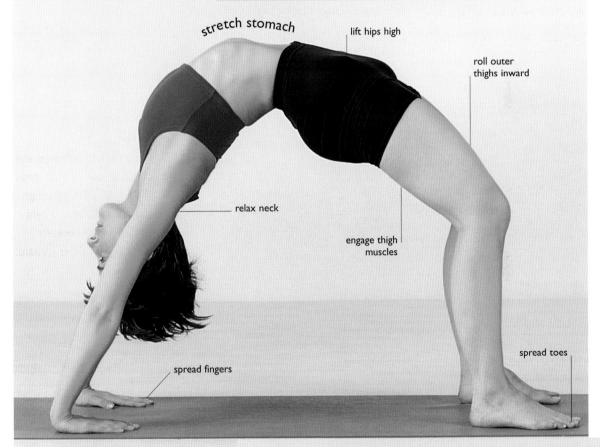

stretch stomach

lift hips high

roll outer thighs inward

relax neck

engage thigh muscles

spread fingers

spread toes

4 Exhaling, lower your hips to the floor, while bending your arms and legs so that you return to the starting position. Rest for several breaths. Repeat the pose one or two times before moving on to the next pose.

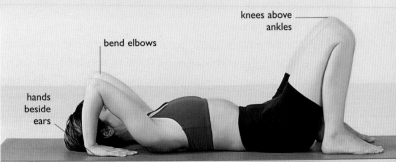

knees above ankles

bend elbows

hands beside ears

URDHVA PRASARITA PADASANA
Upward Extended Foot

This posture strengthens the lower back, tones the abdominal muscles, and is excellent for reducing the waistline. Notice that all movement takes place with the exhale; none with the inhale. There are two key stages to this pose: hold each one for one complete inhalation. Repeat the sequence two to three times.

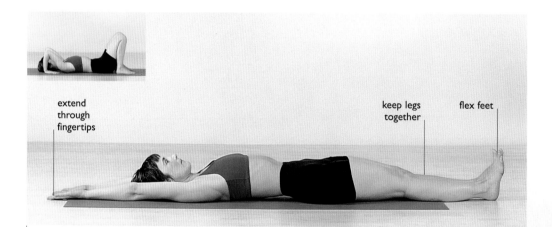

extend through fingertips

keep legs together

flex feet

1 Lying down with your legs bent and your feet flat on the floor, inhale as you reach overhead with your arms, extending the body. Straighten your legs and bring them together. Press through the heels to flex the feet. Gaze forward.

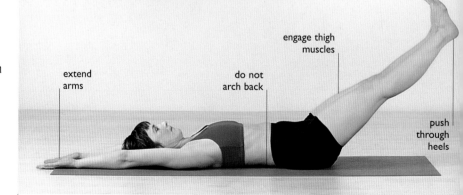

extend arms

do not arch back

engage thigh muscles

push through heels

2 Exhaling, lift your legs halfway up to make a 45° angle and extend the lower back away from the waist and toward the floor. Extend the backs of the legs toward the heels. Hold your legs in this position and take a complete inhalation. Gaze upward.

3 Exhaling, continue to lift your legs to 90°, keeping them firm and together. The soles of the feet should be facing the ceiling. Hold this pose for one complete inhalation. Gaze toward the ceiling.

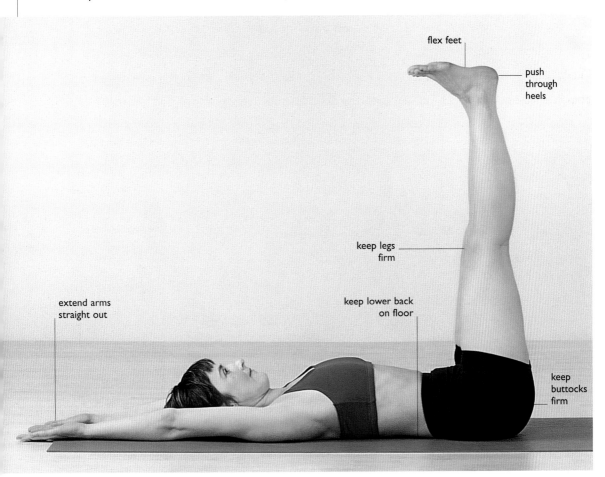

flex feet

push through heels

keep legs firm

extend arms straight out

keep lower back on floor

keep buttocks firm

4 Exhaling, lower both legs together all the way to the floor. Stretch your arms and legs away from each other. Repeat the sequence one or two times more before moving into the next pose.

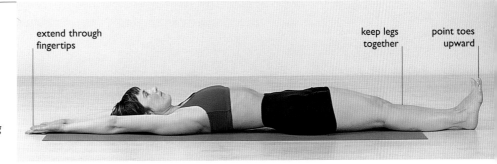

extend through fingertips

keep legs together

point toes upward

JATHARA PARIVARTANASANA
Turning Around the Stomach

This pose allows you to twist the spine and back muscles gently, softening them. It serves as a counterpose to the backward bend poses, preparing the body for the sitting poses. *Jathara parivartasasana* is particularly good if you are feeling tired or stressed as it relaxes you completely. Notice that movement takes place only with the exhale. When you have lowered your legs to both the right and left sides, repeat the entire sequence two more times.

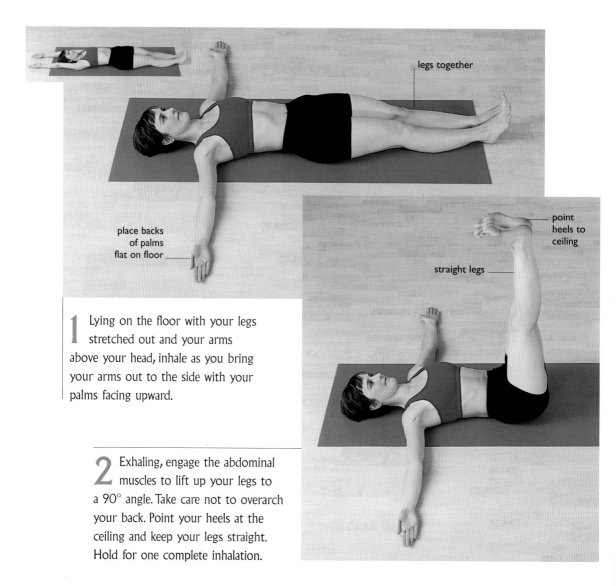

legs together

place backs
of palms
flat on floor

point
heels to
ceiling

straight legs

1 Lying on the floor with your legs stretched out and your arms above your head, inhale as you bring your arms out to the side with your palms facing upward.

2 Exhaling, engage the abdominal muscles to lift up your legs to a 90° angle. Take care not to overarch your back. Point your heels at the ceiling and keep your legs straight. Hold for one complete inhalation.

3 Exhaling, bring your legs down together to the floor on the right side of your body, placing your feet as close to your right hand as possible. Rotate your head to the left. Hold for one complete inhale. Then, exhaling, lift your legs to 90° again, and lower to the left side, rotating your head to the right. Then return to step 1 and repeat two more times.

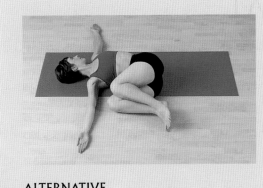

ALTERNATIVE
If you cannot lower both legs together straight, bend them and then lower them to the floor. Place your knees as close to your right arm as possible, while gazing to the left.

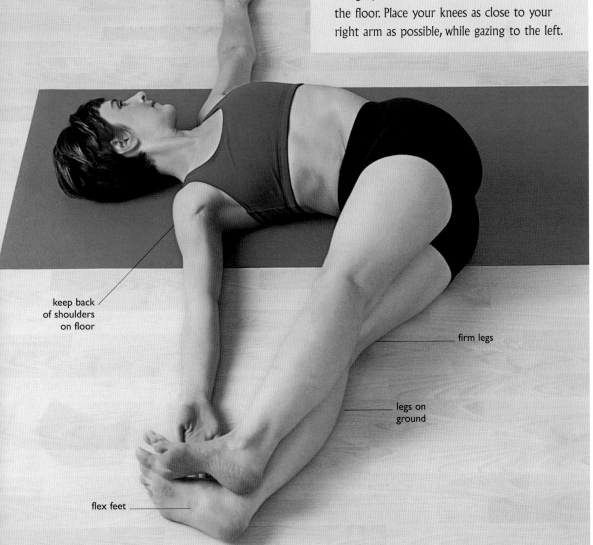

keep back of shoulders on floor

firm legs

legs on ground

flex feet

TRANSITION MOVE
Lying on Back to Sitting

This transitional move is excellent for learning how to use
your body weight and momentum to rock forward to a sitting
position. When done correctly, the move uses very little energy
and helps to tone the abdominal muscles without straining the
lower back muscles.

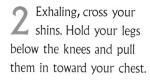

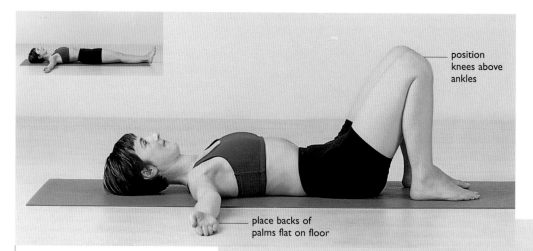

position
knees above
ankles

place backs of
palms flat on floor

1 Lying on your back with
your legs stretched out
straight and your arms at
right angles to the torso,
inhale and bend your knees.
Place your feet flat on the
floor near the buttocks.

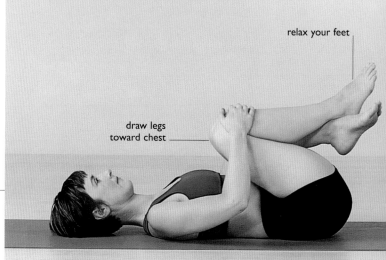

relax your feet

draw legs
toward chest

2 Exhaling, cross your
shins. Hold your legs
below the knees and pull
them in toward your chest.

5 Exhaling, sit up straight, extending the spine and lifting the chest. Rest the outer edge of your feet on the floor and your hands just below the knees. Gaze forward. You are now ready to flow into the next pose.

extend spine

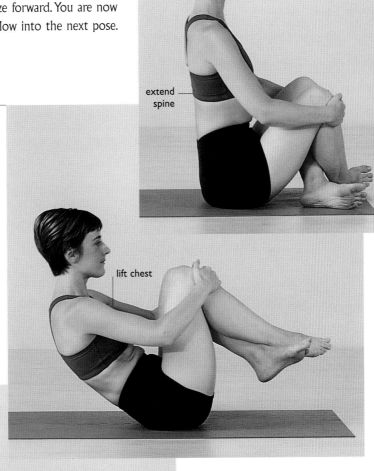

4 Continue inhaling and use the momentum of the rocking motion to roll up onto your sitting bones.

lift chest

3 Inhaling, rock back and lift your middle and lower back off the floor. Pull your legs closer to your chest to form a very tight ball with the body.

lift hips high

ARDHA NAVASANA
Half Boat

In Sanskrit *ardha* means "half" and *nava* "boat," and in this pose the position of the body resembles a boat. It is important not to strain when attempting to do the pose with straight legs. With practice, you will find that your back will strengthen and you will be able to move in and out of the posture gracefully. Hold the pose for five breaths and repeat three times.

1 You are sitting on the floor with your knees up, feet crossed, and hands resting on your knees. Inhale, uncross your feet, and place them flat on the floor. Interlace your fingers and cup the back of the head, keeping the elbows forward. Gaze ahead.

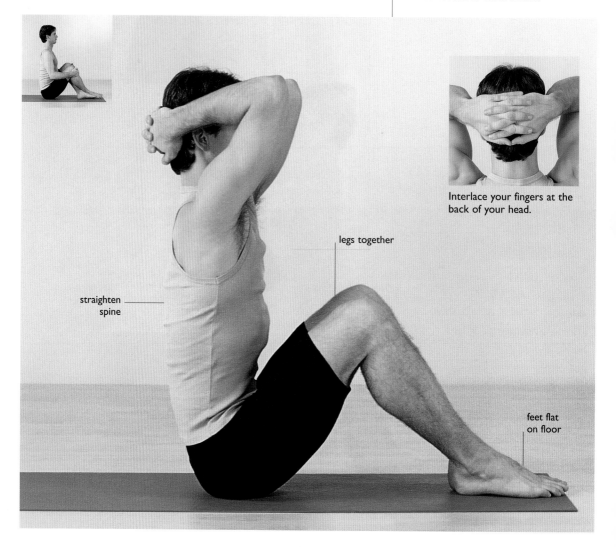

Interlace your fingers at the back of your head.

legs together

straighten spine

feet flat on floor

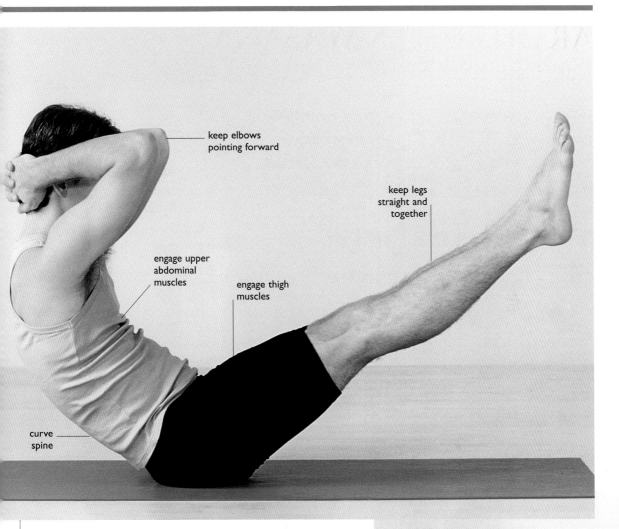

keep elbows
pointing forward

keep legs
straight and
together

engage upper
abdominal
muscles

engage thigh
muscles

curve
spine

2 Exhaling, recline the
torso and simultaneously
lift and straighten your legs.
Rest on your sitting bones,
not on the coccyx. Engage
the abdominal muscles and
keep your head in line with
your toes. Hold the full pose
for five breaths.

3 Inhaling, bend your
knees and lower the feet
to the floor. Place your palms
on the floor by the hips,
with the fingertips pointing
toward the feet. Repeat the
sequence twice more, then
flow into the next pose.

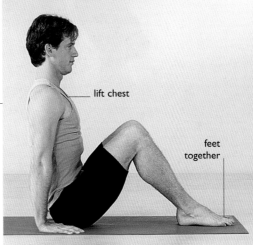

lift chest

feet
together

PARIPURNA NAVASANA
Complete Boat

In Sanskrit *paripurna* means "complete" and *nava* "boat." This posture resembles a boat with its oars in the water, hence "complete boat." It is excellent for reducing fat around the waistline and for toning the kidneys. Hold the full pose for five breaths and repeat three times.

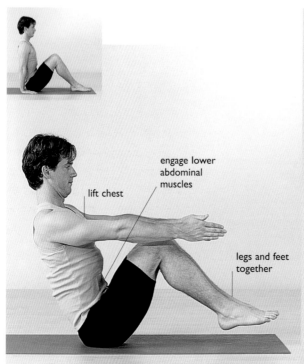

lift chest

engage lower abdominal muscles

legs and feet together

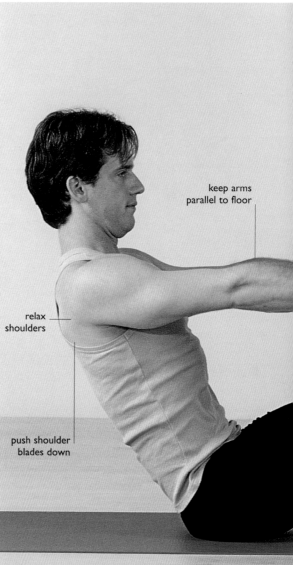

keep arms parallel to floor

relax shoulders

push shoulder blades down

1 Sitting on the floor with your knees up and your arms straight down at your sides, exhale and lean back. Balance on your sitting bones, not the coccyx, and lift your feet off the floor. Extend your arms out in front of you so they are parallel to the floor. Inhale completely.

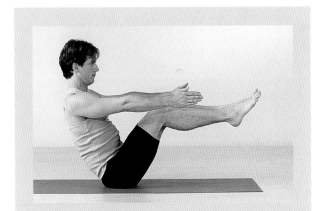

2 Exhaling, straighten your legs by pressing the inner edges of your feet forward. Keep your spine straight and the chest lifted. Gaze at your big toes. Hold *Paripurna navasana* for five breaths.

ALTERNATIVE
If you find that your back and abdominal muscles are not strong enough to keep the spine straight in the full pose, bend your knees. Make sure you still keep your legs together.

3 Exhaling, lower your feet to the floor and bend your knees. Move your arms to your sides, palms down, and press your hands into the mat. Repeat the sequence twice more, then move to the next pose.

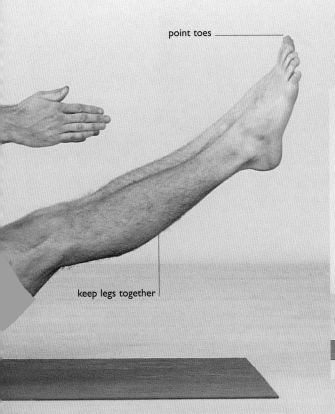

point toes

keep legs together

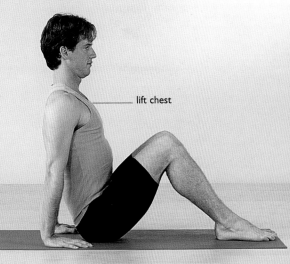

lift chest

BAKASANA
Crane

In Sanskrit *baka* means "crane." Once the legs are lifted, this posture resembles a crane standing still. The pose is excellent for building strength in the arms and abdomen. It also develops courage, because to do the pose you have to overcome fear and believe that you can balance and not fall forward. Hold the pose for five breaths and repeat twice.

2 Exhaling, pull the feet close to the buttocks. Rock the body forward, lifting the buttocks off the floor and shifting the weight forward on the feet. Keep just the tips of your fingers touching the floor. Gaze slightly downward.

1 Sitting on the floor with your knees up and your palms on the floor, inhale and lean slightly forward. Bend your arms and lift your hands, so that only your fingertips are touching the floor.

tips of fingers on floor

keep feet flat on floor

feet wide apart

fingertips on floor

3 Inhaling, bring your arms forward and place your hands flat on the floor in front of you, fingers spread and pointing forward. Press the knees into the back of your arms near the armpits. Bend the arms to create a stable support for the legs.

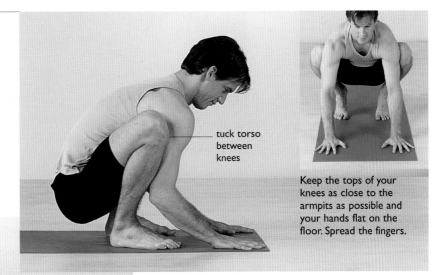

tuck torso between knees

Keep the tops of your knees as close to the armpits as possible and your hands flat on the floor. Spread the fingers.

4 Exhaling, raise the heels high off the floor, shifting the weight forward onto your hands. Balance the shins on your bent arms as close to the armpits as possible. Gaze at the floor.

5 Continue exhaling and engage *mula bandha*. Swing your body forward and pull the feet toward the buttocks. Straighten your arms and balance the entire weight of your body on your hands. Hold the pose for five breaths. Repeat the sequence once more, then move straight into the next pose.

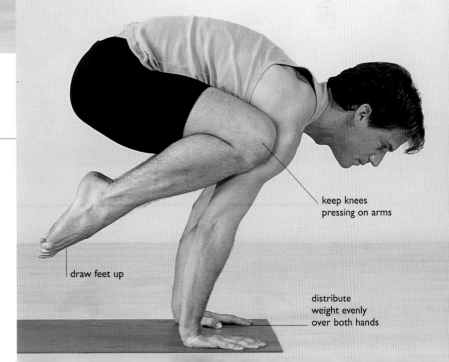

keep knees pressing on arms

draw feet up

distribute weight evenly over both hands

TRANSITION MOVE
Crane to Sitting

Here is another transition from one pose to another integrating several movements from the Sun Salutations, which should by now be quite familiar. Be patient when doing this transition: it takes a lot of practice to develop the ability to move your body while balancing on just your hands.

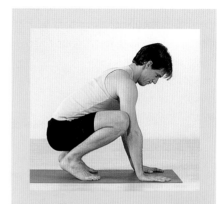

1 Starting from the Crane position (*p.107*), exhale as you push off your arms, propelling the feet back and extending your legs parallel to the floor in mid-air. Land on the balls of your feet in the push-up position. Gaze downward.

ALTERNATIVE
If you cannot jump your feet back and extend your legs in mid-air, then lower both feet to the floor in a squat, and step back one leg at a time into the push-up position.

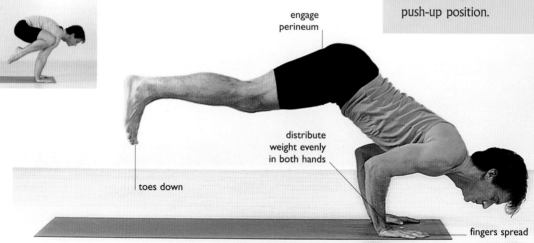

engage perineum

distribute weight evenly in both hands

toes down

fingers spread

whole sequence at a glance

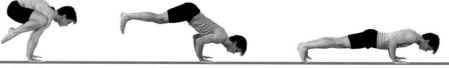

Inhaling.................Begin exhaling...................Finish exhaling..........

2 Continue exhaling as you lower your body evenly until it is 4–6in (10–15cm) above, and parallel to, the floor in *Chaturanga dhandasana (p.32)*. Keep your arms bent with the elbows in very close to the sides of your torso. Gaze at the floor.

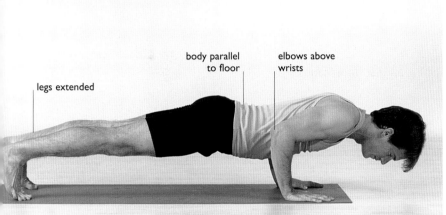

legs extended

body parallel to floor

elbows above wrists

3 Inhaling, roll forward onto the tops of your feet into *Urdhva mukha svanasana (p.32)*. Straighten your arms, pull your hips forward, and lift up the chest so your whole body is lifted off the floor. Keep the legs firm.

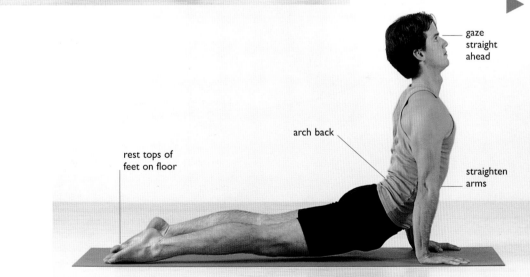

gaze straight ahead

arch back

rest tops of feet on floor

straighten arms

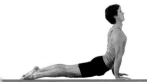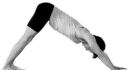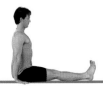

.........Inhaling.................Exhaling, then inhaling...........Exhaling..................Inhaling

4 Exhaling, lift your hips up and back, pushing the sitting bones toward the ceiling into *Adho mukha svanasana* (*p.33*). Push through the roots of your fingers to straighten the arms, and push back with your legs so the soles of your feet are flat on the floor. Spread your weight evenly on your hands and feet. Keep your head in line with the torso. Gaze back. Inhale completely.

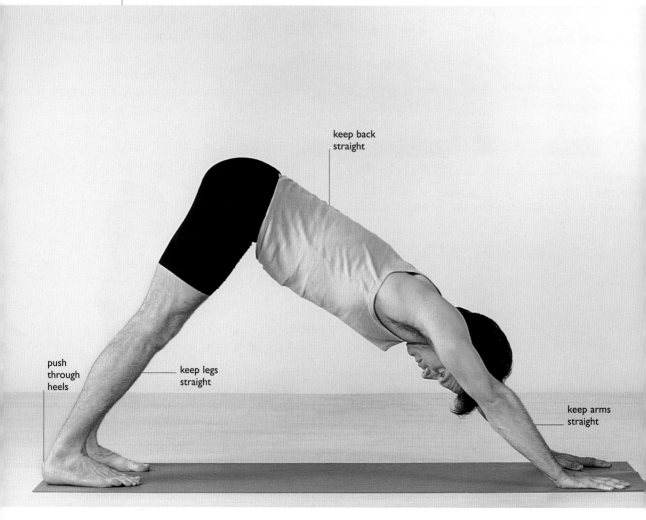

keep back
straight

push
through
heels

keep legs
straight

keep arms
straight

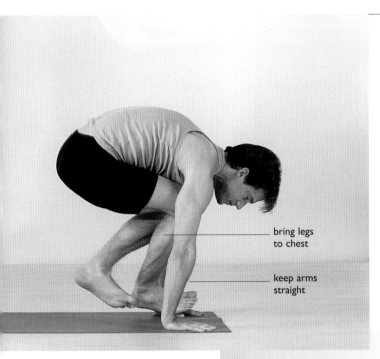

bring legs
to chest

keep arms
straight

5 Exhaling, bend your knees and push off the floor with your feet, crossing your legs in mid-air and compacting the torso into a crouching position. Keep the feet off the floor as the legs are propelled through the arms and then straightened. The legs and the buttocks will land on the floor in front of the torso at the same time. If you cannot swing through to sitting in one movement, do the move in two stages: let your crossed feet rest on the mat as they come between your arms (*see p.91*), and then move them forward in front of your torso and straighten.

6 Take an inhalation in the final position. The legs are extended forward and the arms straight at your sides. The hands point forward and toes upward. Gaze straight ahead. You are now ready to move into the next pose.

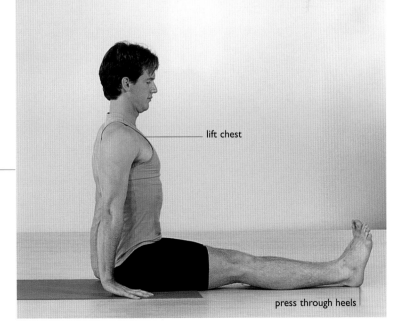

lift chest

press through heels

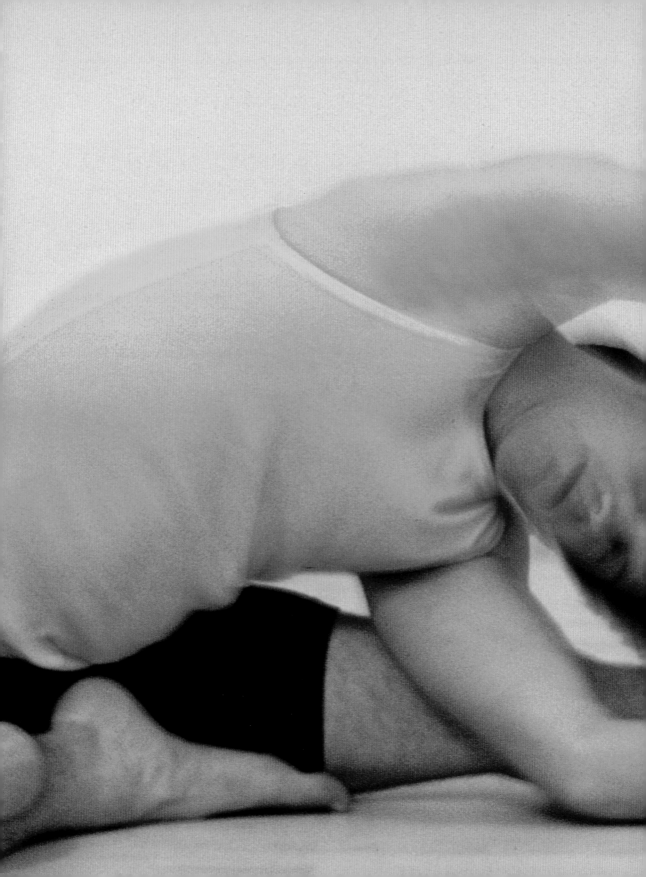

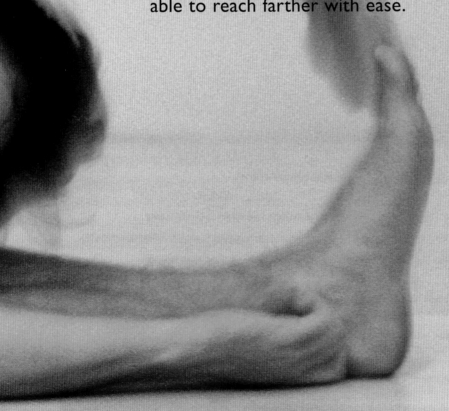

SEATED POSES

After the backward bends we now slow the rhythm
a little with a sequence of seated poses. With these
it is important to maintain proper alignment and to
avoid the tendency to constrict your chest in an
effort to reach farther. To begin with, it is common
to feel tightness throughout the hips and hamstrings,
limiting your movement in these *asanas*. Do not
become discouraged: with practice you will be
able to reach farther with ease.

JANU SIRSASANA
Knee to Head

This pose is excellent for the digestive system and also helps
tone the kidneys. After holding the pose on the right side for
five to eight breaths, it is best to keep the right leg bent and
carry straight on to the next pose, *Parivrtta janu sirsasana*
(*pp.116–117*), before changing to the left side of the body.
Then repeat both poses in sequence on the left side.

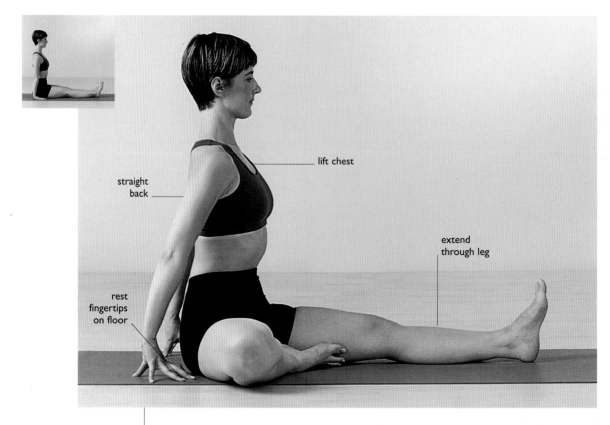

lift chest

straight
back

extend
through leg

rest
fingertips
on floor

1 Sitting on the floor with your legs out straight
in front and your arms down by your sides, inhale
and bend your right knee to the side to make a 90°
angle. Position the heel as close as possible to the
perineum. Push up with your hands so that only
the fingertips are resting on the floor.

2 Exhaling, lean forward, and grasp the
wrist of your right hand with your left
hand behind the extended foot. Inhaling, fold
your body forward, bending your elbows, so
that your chest rests on your left leg and
your forehead on your shin. Keep the sitting
bones rooted to the floor. Gaze forward.
Hold for five to eight breaths, then inhale
and sit upright in the step 1 position ready
to move into *Parivrtta janu sirsasana* (*pp.116–117*).

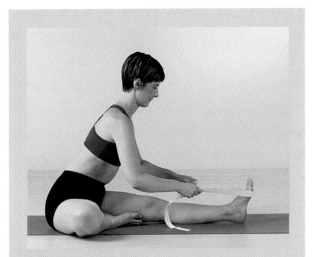

ALTERNATIVE

If you cannot reach far enough forward without
bending your extended leg, place a strap underneath
the ball of your foot. Pull on the strap, working
your hands closer to the foot. Keep your sitting
bones grounded and your spine lengthened.

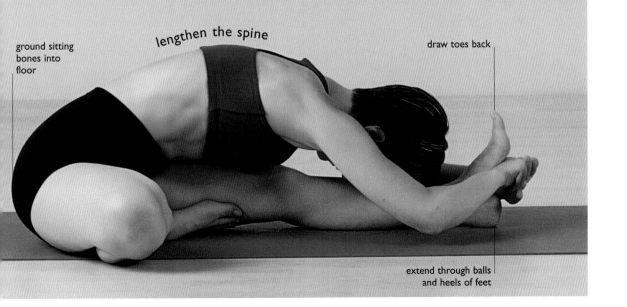

lengthen the spine

ground sitting
bones into
floor

draw toes back

extend through balls
and heels of feet

PARIVRTTA JANU SIRSASANA
Revolving Knee to Head

This pose is similar to the previous one, but here the torso revolves as the head moves toward the knee. It is a very invigorating pose, which stimulates the circulation. Hold the full pose for five to eight breaths, then go back to step 1 of *janu sirsasana (pp.114–115)*, and repeat the entire sequence on the left side of the body.

1 Sitting on the floor, your right knee bent, heel tucked into the perineum, inhale and turn the torso and hips to the right. Extend your right knee back while keeping your right foot near the groin. Move your arms to the front.

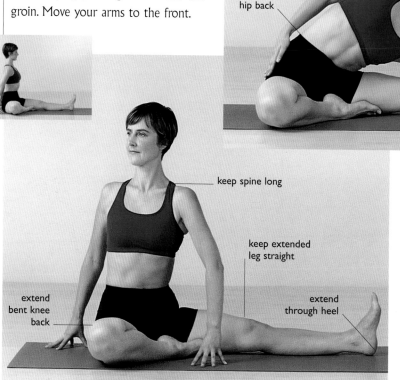

rotate hip back

keep arm inside leg

keep spine long

keep extended leg straight

extend bent knee back

extend through heel

2 Exhaling, extend the torso over the left leg while stretching your right side and rotating the right rib cage upward. Keep the right heel close to the pubic bone. Grab hold of the arch of your left foot with your left hand. Gaze up.

If you cannot reach your extended foot with both hands, place your left hand on the floor by the extended foot and the right hand on the back of the neck. It is more important to lengthen the waist and spine than to grab the foot.

3 Inhaling, extend your right hand up and over to grab hold of the outside of your left foot. Press the sitting bones into the mat and lift the waist. Gaze up. Hold the pose for five to eight breaths. Exhale and return to step 1 of *Janu sirsasana* (*p.114*) to repeat both poses on the other side.

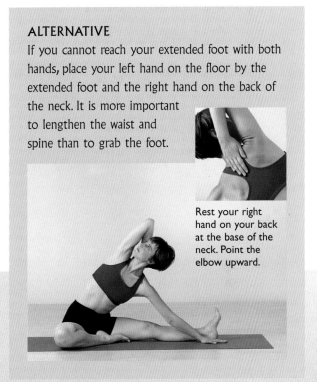

Rest your right hand on your back at the base of the neck. Point the elbow upward.

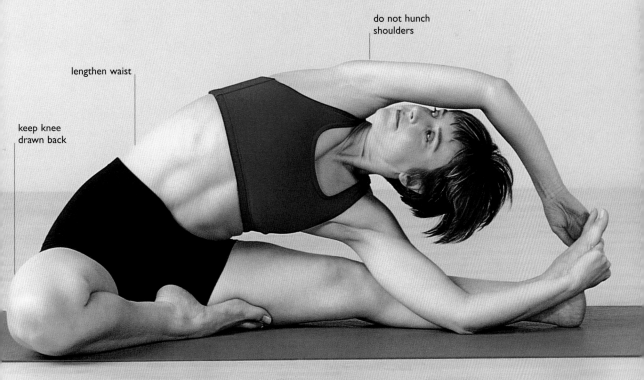

do not hunch shoulders

lengthen waist

keep knee drawn back

ARDHA BADDHA PADMA PASCHIMATTANASANA
Half Bound Lotus Forward Bend

Paschimattanasana is a posterior stretch. This pose, which should not be forced, is good for rounded or drooping shoulders. Make sure you open your hips before resting the foot near the groin; otherwise, you can damage the knee. Hold this pose for five to eight breaths on the right side of the body, then go straight on to the following pose, *Ardha matsyendrasana* (*pp.120–121*), and do that on the same side before repeating both poses on the left side of the body.

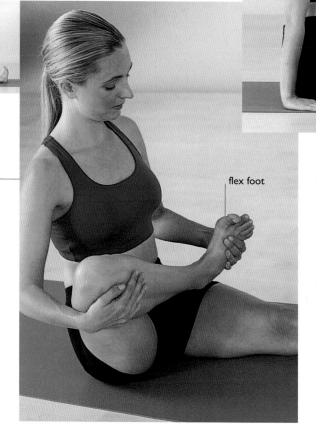

rest foot on thigh close to body

face knee upward

flex foot

1 Sit on the floor with your legs out straight in front and your arms down at your sides. Place your palms on the floor, fingers pointing forward. Inhaling, grab the outside of your right knee and the right foot. Place the foot on top of the left thigh close to the groin. Turn the pelvis so the right knee faces forward.

2 Continue inhaling. Sit up very straight with your hands flat on the floor and close to your hips. Press the inner edge of your left foot forward. Gaze at your left big toe.

3 Exhaling, reach around your back with your right arm to grasp your right foot. Begin to fold forward, creating a twisting action in the hips. Grasp your left foot with the left hand, and gaze downward. Hold for five to eight breaths. Inhale to return to step 2 ready to flow into *Ardha matsyendrasana* (pp.120–121).

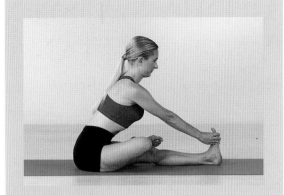

ALTERNATIVE

If your hips are very tight and you are unable to lean far enough forward, place your right foot just above your left knee and reach for your left foot with both hands.

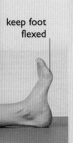

keep foot flexed

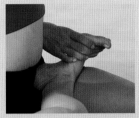

Reach around your back with your right hand and grab hold of your right foot. Keep the foot flexed and do not allow the ankle to collapse inward.

draw down shoulders away from ears

keep chest open

rotate thigh bone inward

ARDHA MATSYENDRASANA
Half Lord of the Fish

In Sanskrit *ardha* means "half," and Matsyendra was a fish transformed by Siva into a divine being who would spread the teaching of yoga. If you have a spinal injury, seek the guidance of an experienced teacher before doing any twist postures. This pose, held for five to eight breaths, is done in conjunction with the previous pose, *Ardha baddha padma paschimattanasana.*

1 Sitting on the floor, your right knee bent, heel tucked close to the pubic bone, inhale and turn to your left, placing your right hand on the left shin. Sit up very straight, draw in the sacrum, and lengthen the spine. Keep the chest lifted. Gaze ahead.

2 Exhaling, wrap your left arm around your back and lean toward your extended leg. Grab hold of your inner right thigh with your left hand.

draw shoulders down

extend through ball and heel of foot

keep foot flexed

ground sitting bones

3 Inhaling, grab the outer edge of your left foot with your right hand and lift and turn the torso to the left. Pull against your right foot to increase the twist. Gaze over your left shoulder. Hold the full pose for five to eight breaths. Then exhale and sit in *Dandasana* ready to begin the entire sequence again on the other side of the body (*p.118*).

ALTERNATIVE

If you cannot reach your inner thigh with your left hand, rest the back of your hand on the outside of your right buttock. Turn your body to the left while holding the left foot.

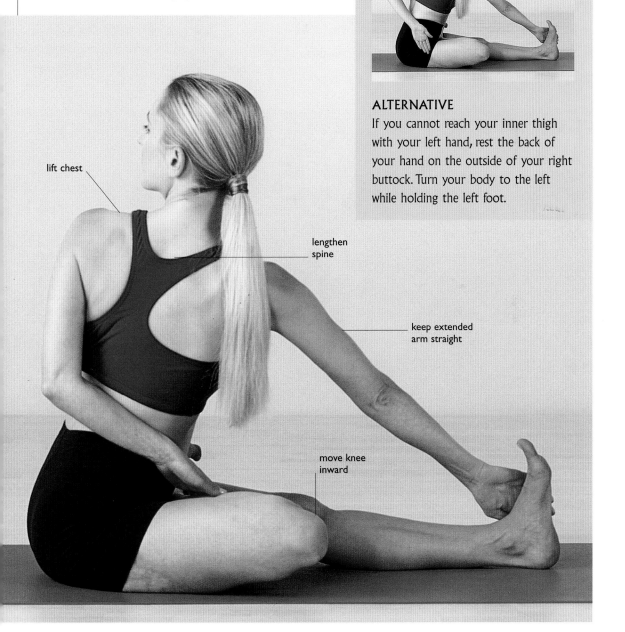

lift chest

lengthen spine

keep extended arm straight

move knee inward

MARICHYASANA A
Marichi A

The following series of postures are named after Marichi, the mythical sage and son of Brahma, creator of the universe. They are excellent for the digestive system. Hold this posture on the right side for five to eight breaths, then do the next posture, *Marichyasana C,* on the same side. Once both poses are completed on the right side, do both on the left.

2 Exhaling, reach forward with your right arm, lowering and extending the torso toward your left leg. Place your right shoulder as low as possible in front of your right shin. Reaching with the right hand helps extend the torso and spine. Press through your right foot.

1 Sit in *Dandasana,* with your legs out straight in front, your arms at your sides. Inhaling, bend your right leg and place your right foot in front of your right sitting bone. Move your hands back behind you and sit up straight, extending through the left foot. Gaze forward.

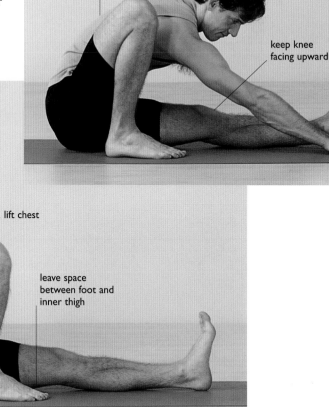

extend spine

keep knee facing upward

lift chest

leave space between foot and inner thigh

lengthen spine

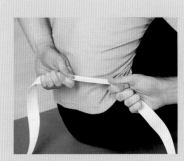

ALTERNATIVE
If you cannot reach the wrist or fingers of your left hand, hold a strap in both hands behind your back. Position your hands as close to each other as you can.

Spread the fingers of your left hand wide as you hold your wrist.

relax shoulders down

draw sitting bones toward the floor

press evenly through ball and heel of foot

press back of knee to floor

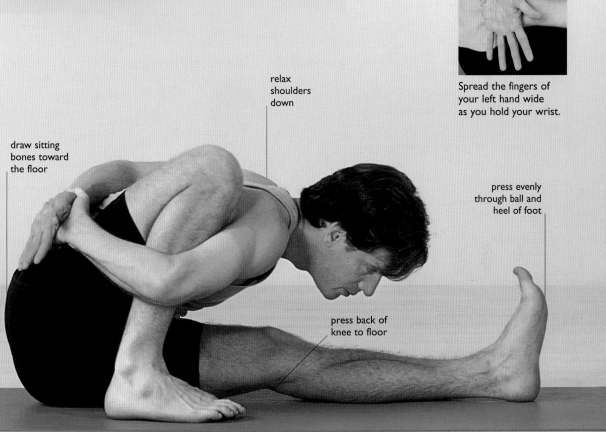

3 Continue exhaling and wrap your right arm around your back and grab your left wrist. Lower your chin toward the left shin, keeping the right foot grounded evenly on the floor. Spread the toes. Keep the right sitting bone as low to the floor as possible. Gaze down at the floor. Hold *Marichyasana A* for five to eight breaths. Then inhale and return to the pose in step 1, ready for *Marichyasana C* (pp.124–125).

MARICHYASANA C
Marichi C

This pose and the previous pose, *Marichyasana A,* are both good
for relieving menstrual cramps and strengthening the uterus, as
well as helping with stomach and gastrointestinal problems.
Hold the pose for five to eight breaths on the right side, then
return to *Marichyasana A (pp.122–123),* change legs, and repeat
the entire sequence on the left side.

1 Sit on the floor with your left leg
extended and the right foot in front
of the sitting bones. Inhaling, rotate the
torso to the right by pressing your left
heel forward and pushing down evenly
on your right foot.

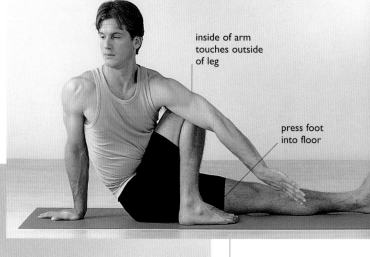

inside of arm
touches outside
of leg

press foot
into floor

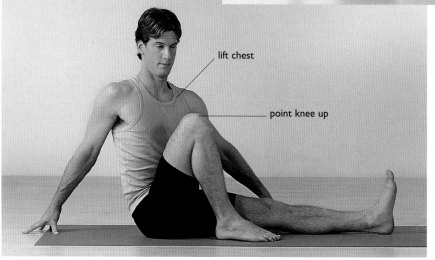

lift chest

point knee up

2 Exhaling, bring
your right arm
closer to the torso and
press your palm into
the floor. Wrap your
left arm around the
outside of your right
leg. Push both sitting
bones into the floor.
Rotate your left arm
so the inside is
touching the outside
of your right leg.

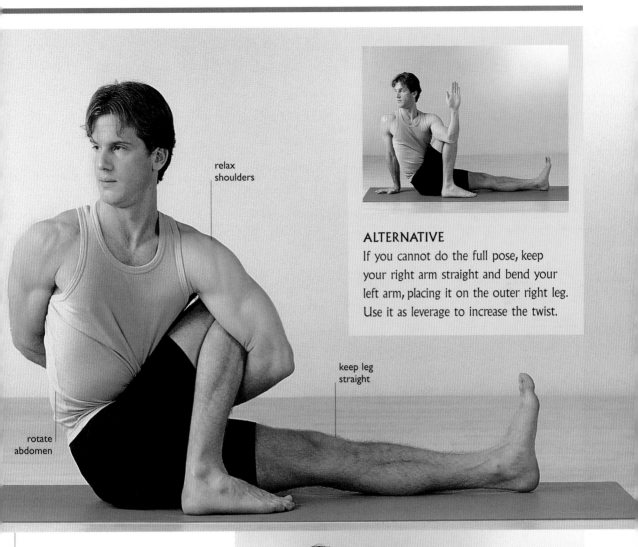

relax
shoulders

rotate
abdomen

keep leg
straight

ALTERNATIVE
If you cannot do the full pose, keep
your right arm straight and bend your
left arm, placing it on the outer right leg.
Use it as leverage to increase the twist.

3 Inhaling, extend your right arm
behind your back and grab
hold of your left wrist. Relax your
shoulders down and lift the chest.
Gaze at a point on the horizon, and
hold for five to eight breaths.

4 Exhaling, release your arms and
straighten your right leg. Sit up
tall in Dandasana in preparation for
Marichyasana A (pp.122–123) on the left
side. To finish, remain in this position
ready for the next pose.

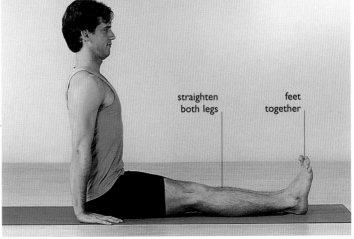

straighten
both legs

feet
together

PASCHIMATTANASANA
Seated Forward Bend

In Sanskrit *paschima* means "the west," and in this pose the back of the body is referred to as the western aspect and the front as the eastern aspect. This asana, which stretches the western aspect, is calming and helps to deepen the breath and engage *mula bandha.* Hold the pose for five to eight breaths.

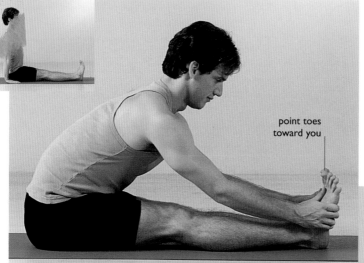

point toes
toward you

2 Inhaling, lift the torso, pulling back on your feet while pushing the balls and heels evenly forward. Straighten the spine and lift the chest.

1 Sitting on the floor with your legs out straight in front of you and your arms at your sides, exhale and fold your body forward at the hips to grab the outer edges of your feet. Keep your legs straight and extend through the four corners of your feet, pressing the back of your knees to the floor. Gaze at your big toes.

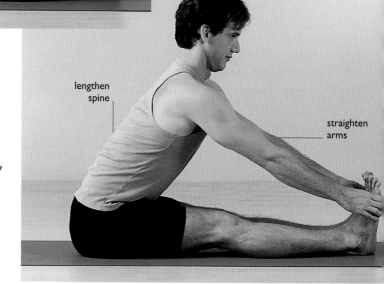

lengthen
spine

straighten
arms

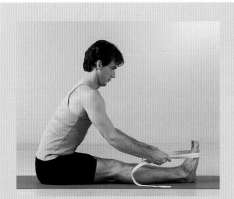

ALTERNATIVE

If you cannot reach the outer edges of your feet, wrap a strap under the balls of your feet and hold each end. As you push forward with your heels and balls of the feet, pull back on the strap with both hands.

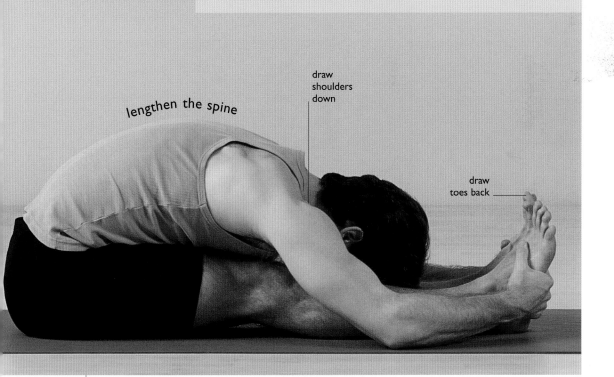

lengthen the spine

draw
shoulders
down

draw
toes back

3 Exhaling, fold all the way forward, extending the front of your body over your legs and holding the outside edge of both feet. Lengthen the waist and push the sitting bones into the floor. Rotate your thighs slightly inward, keeping your legs straight and firm. Hold the full pose for five to eight breaths. Then inhale and return to *Dandasana*, ready for the next pose.

BADDHA KONASANA
Bound Angle

This posture is wonderful for relieving menstrual cramps and an excellent prenatal pose. It also helps with urinary disorders and can alleviate symptoms of sciatica. Do not force the knees down to the floor, and let the groin open naturally. If you suffer from knee pain, place folded blankets under each leg for support. Hold for five to eight breaths.

1 Sit on the floor with your legs out straight in front of you and your arms at your sides. Inhaling, fold your legs in, and use your hands to bring the heels together next to the groin. Roll the pelvis so the sitting bones are pressing straight down. Engage *mula* and *uddiyana bandha*. Gaze forward.

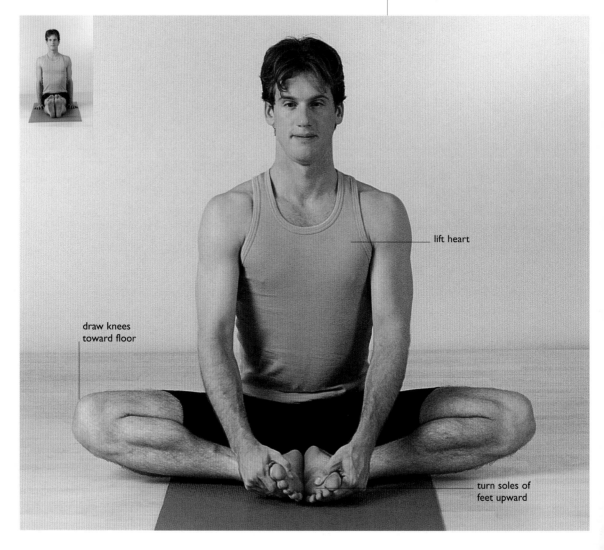

lift heart

draw knees
toward floor

turn soles of
feet upward

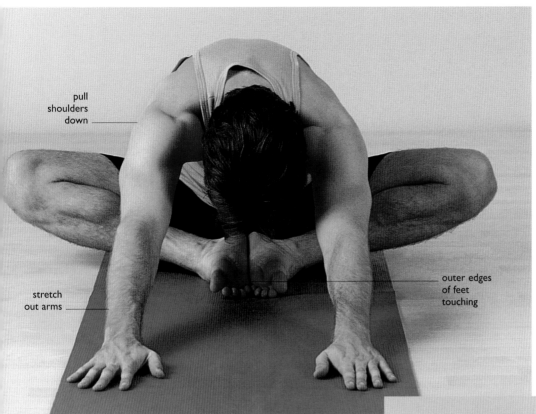

pull
shoulders
down

stretch
out arms

outer edges
of feet
touching

2 Exhaling, fold the body forward from the hips into *Baddha konasana.* Keep the sitting bones pressed to the floor. Release the feet and reach forward with your arms, stretching out the fingertips. Lengthen the spine, creating space between each vertebrae. Keep your heels and knees down. Gaze at the floor. Hold for five to eight breaths.

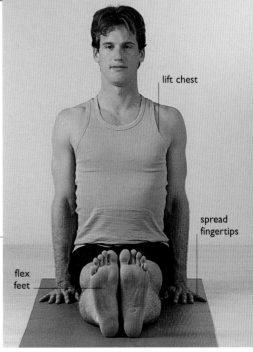

lift chest

spread
fingertips

flex
feet

3 Inhaling, lift your torso up straight and extend your legs parallel in front of you. Place your hands on the floor beside your hips with fingertips facing forward. Flex your feet and gaze straight ahead, and get ready for the next pose.

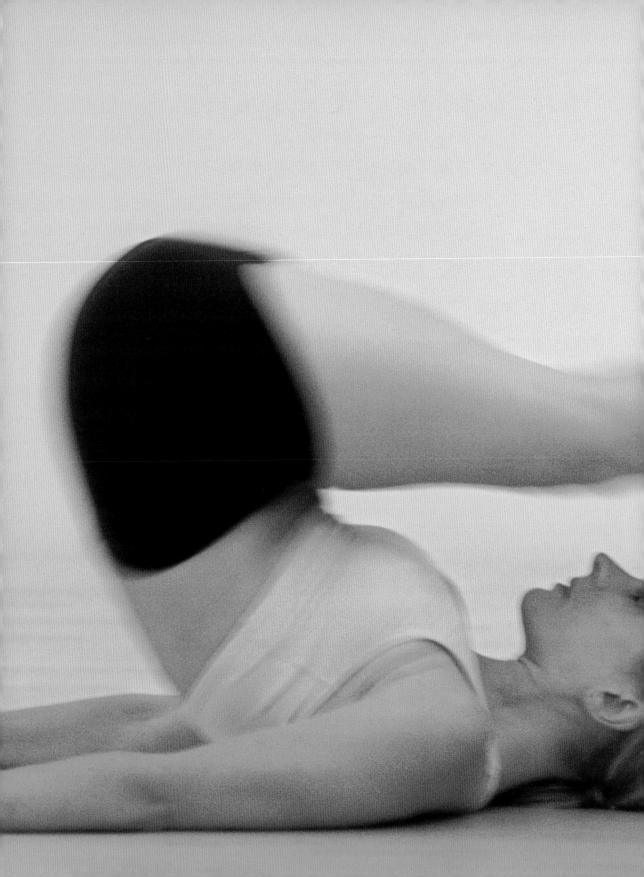

INVERTED POSES

Apprehension is the greatest obstacle you will face in practicing this sequence of inverted postures. Their challenging nature demands that you push your body to the limit of its ability without causing injury. This is known as "playing your edge." I cannot overemphasize the importance of moving with intention and remaining completely focused throughout each of the poses in this section.

SALAMBA SIRSASANA & BALASANA
Headstand & Child's pose

The headstand is considered the king of all poses. When you stand on your head, the blood flows to the brain and the mind becomes alert and clear. It is a wonderful antidote for insomnia and headaches. However, if you have high blood pressure or a cervical spine injury, it is best to consult a qualified teacher before trying this pose. Hold the pose for at least 25 breaths.

1 Get onto all fours with knees hip-width apart and hands shoulder-width apart. Exhaling, lower the crown of your head and your forearms to the floor. Interlace your fingers and place the outer edges of your hands on the floor. Draw in the elbows so they align with the shoulders.

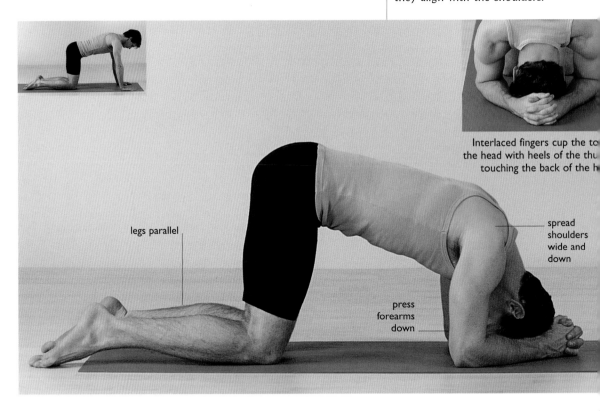

Interlaced fingers cup the to the head with heels of the thu touching the back of the h

legs parallel

spread shoulders wide and down

press forearms down

whole sequence at a glance

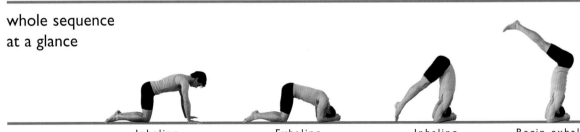

Inhaling................Exhaling................Inhaling............Begin exhali

2 Inhaling, distribute your body weight
evenly onto the forearms. Engage both
mula and *uddiyana bandhas.* Straighten your legs
and slowly walk your feet toward your face,
shifting the hips back. Gaze toward your feet.

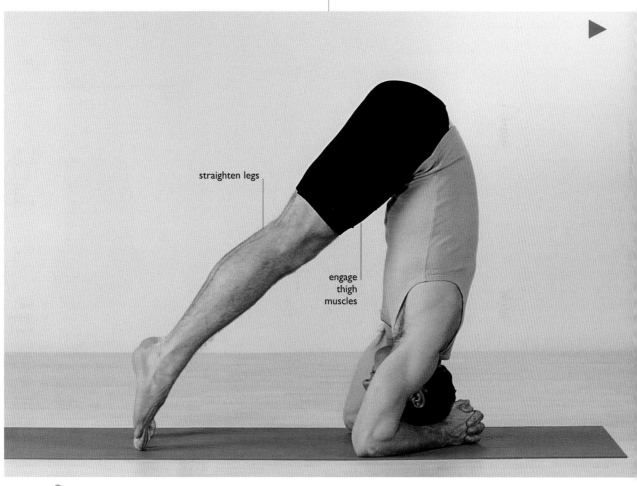

straighten legs

engage
thigh
muscles

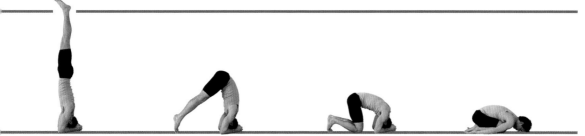

Finish exhaling and inhale...........Exhaling.....................Inhaling.................Exhaling

3 Exhaling, lift your legs into the air. Shift your hips back farther than your hands, so that your weight is resting on the forearms evenly. Gaze straight ahead.

4 Continue exhaling and extend the inner edges of the feet to the ceiling, straightening your legs into the full pose. Pull the shoulder blades firmly down the back and lengthen the back of the neck. Continue to press down through the forearms and sides of the hands. Gaze upward. Hold the headstand for at least 25 breaths.

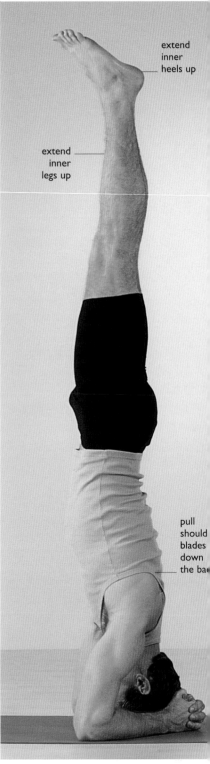

extend inner heels up

extend inner legs up

pull should blades down the ba

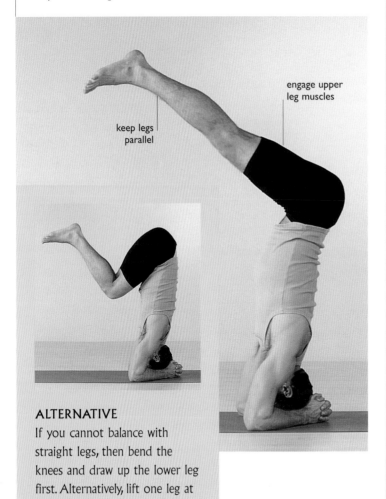

keep legs parallel

engage upper leg muscles

ALTERNATIVE

If you cannot balance with straight legs, then bend the knees and draw up the lower leg first. Alternatively, lift one leg at a time. You may find it helpful to begin by doing the headstand against a wall.

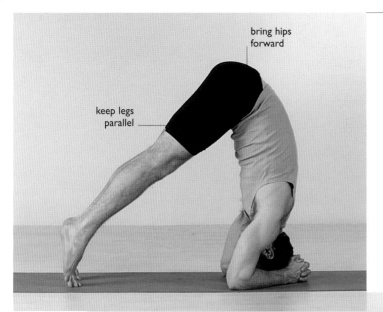

bring hips forward

keep legs parallel

5 Exhaling, slowly lower your feet to the floor, shifting your hips forward. Keep your legs together and straight as you bring your toes to the floor. Gaze at your feet.

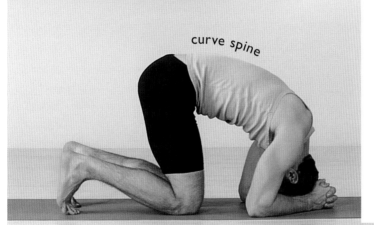

curve spine

6 Inhale as the balls of your feet touch the floor. Bend your legs and lower the knees to the floor in a crouching position. Rest feet on curled-under toes.

7 Exhaling, unlace your fingers and bring your arms to the sides of your legs with the palms facing upward. Lower your hips so your legs are folded. Place your forehead on the floor and rest in child's pose, *Balasana,* until all tension is released in the shoulders and neck. When you are ready, sit up straight, ready for the next pose.

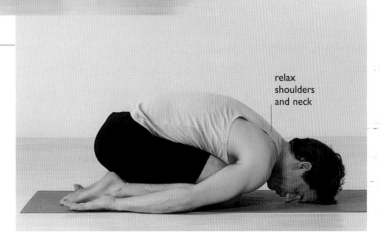

relax shoulders and neck

SALAMBA SARVANGASANA
Shoulder stand

If the headstand is considered the king of poses, the shoulder stand is considered the queen. In Sanskrit *sarvanga* means "entire body," and the whole body does indeed benefit from the shoulder stand. This pose improves the circulation and breathing, and relieves constipation. Hold the pose for at least 25 breaths. Then move straight on to the plow and ear pressure poses shown on the next two pages.

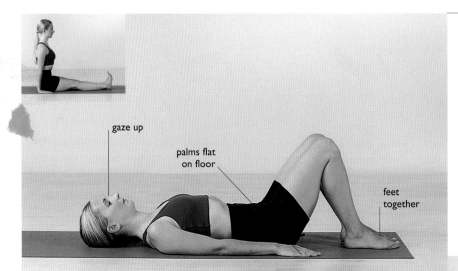

gaze up

palms flat on floor

feet together

1 Sit on the floor with your legs out straight in front of you. Exhaling, lay down on your back. Bend the knees and draw your legs up, placing your feet flat on the floor and together. Rest your arms by the side of the body. Inhale.

2 Exhaling, press your hands into the floor and lift the bent legs and hips up in the air. Straighten the legs as your feet reach over your head.

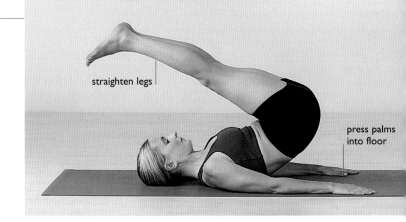

straighten legs

press palms into floor

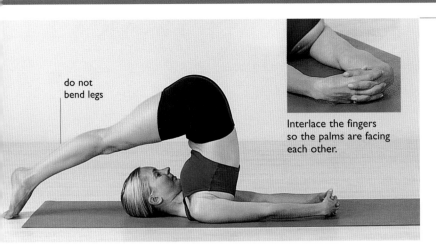

do not
bend legs

Interlace the fingers
so the palms are facing
each other.

3 Inhaling, extend your
legs so the tips of your
toes touch the floor. Keep
the legs very straight and
firm. Bring your hands
together, interlacing your
fingers. Keep your arms
straight and firm. Walk the
shoulders in and draw the
elbows close to each other.

4 Exhaling, place the
palms of your hands
on the middle back
without moving the
elbows outward. Point
your fingertips toward
the ceiling. Bend the
knees and lift them up,
folding your legs in half.
Inhale completely.

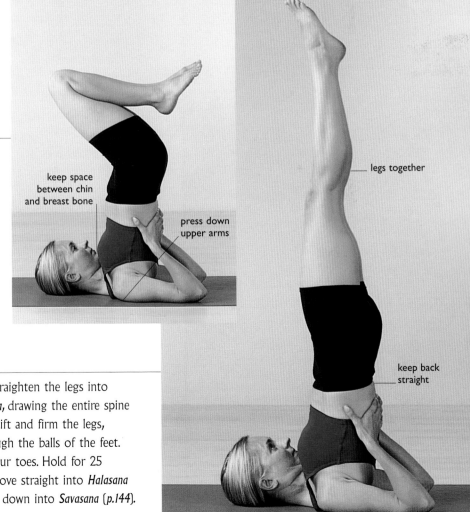

keep space
between chin
and breast bone

press down
upper arms

legs together

keep back
straight

5 Exhaling, straighten the legs into
Sarvangasana, drawing the entire spine
into the body. Lift and firm the legs,
extending through the balls of the feet.
Gaze toward your toes. Hold for 25
breaths. Then move straight into *Halasana*
(*p.138*), or come down into *Savasana* (*p.144*).

HALASANA & KARNAPIDASANA
Plow & Ear Pressure Pose

The shape made by the body in the first of these poses, *Halasana*, resembles a plow, hence its name. Both *Halasana* and *Karnapidasana* rejuvenate the abdominal organs and can help relieve backache. In Sanskrit *karna* means "ear" and *pida* means "pressure." Hold each pose for five to eight breaths.

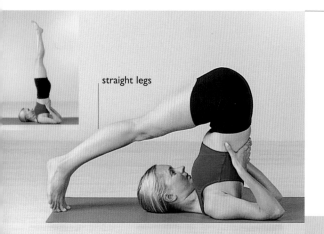

straight legs

1 From the shoulder stand position move into *Halasana.* Exhaling, lower your feet over your head until your toes touch the floor. Extend through the heels, firming and straightening the legs. Hold the pose for five to eight breaths.

2 Now move into *Karnapidasana.* Exhaling, bend your legs and place your knees next to your ears if you can. Rest the tops of your feet on the floor. Bring your arms out straight and place on the floor above you. Interlace your fingers. Gaze forward. Hold for five to eight breaths.

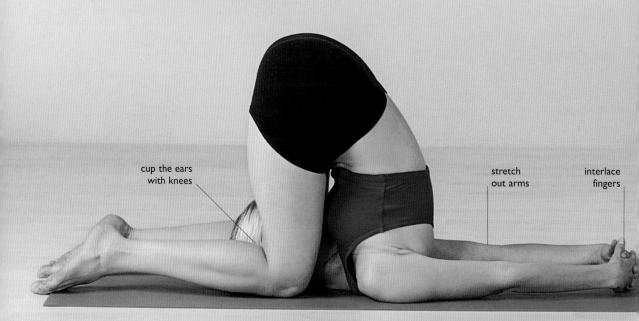

cup the ears with knees

stretch out arms

interlace fingers

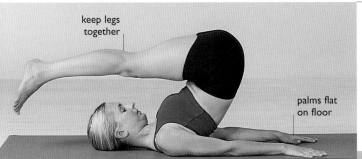

keep legs together

palms flat on floor

3 Exhaling, release the hands and press your palms firmly into the floor. Straighten your legs, lifting them off the floor. Gradually lower the hips to the floor, engaging the abdominal and thigh muscles.

legs parallel

4 At the end of the exhale, bring your legs right down to the floor. Inhaling, relax the entire body as you lie flat on the floor for several breaths. Gaze upward.

5 Exhaling, raise your legs from the floor and clasp your knees with your hands. Pull your knees toward your chest. Make sure the lower region of the spine remains in contact with the floor and draw the shoulders down the back.

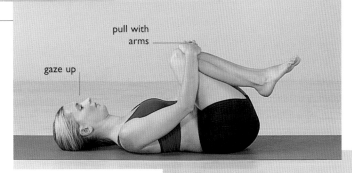

pull with arms

gaze up

6 Inhaling, cross your legs at the shins and rock up to a sitting position, still holding your knees. Sit up straight with both feet flat on the floor. Lengthen the spine, extending through the crown of the head. Prepare to extend your legs for *Padmasana 1 (pp.140–141)*.

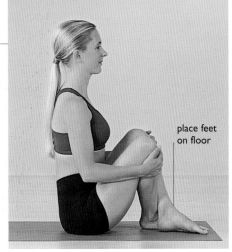

place feet on floor

PADMASANA 1
Lotus 1

The lotus is the posture of meditation and most commonly associated with yoga. It has several variants of varying degrees of difficulty. Start by doing only the version shown here. Then, when you are comfortable with it, move on to also do the more advanced version shown on pages 142–143. If you have very stiff hips or feel any pinching or discomfort in the knees, do the alternative to the full pose. Hold the full pose for 10 breaths.

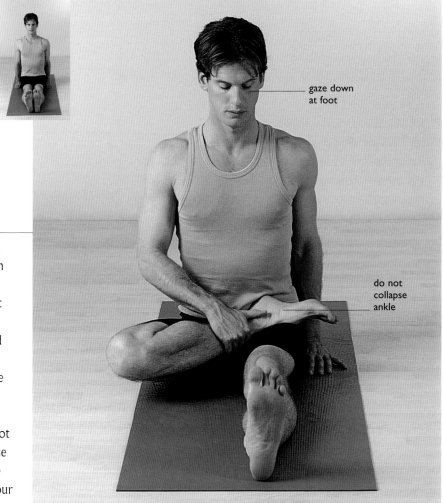

gaze down at foot

do not collapse ankle

1 Inhaling, sit up straight, arms by your sides, with your legs out straight in front of you and your feet flexed. Grasp your right ankle with your right hand and fold your right leg in toward your belly. Place the right foot on top of the upper left thigh. Keep the right foot flexed and do not allow the inner ankle of the right leg to collapse. Move your right arm back by your side, palm on the floor.

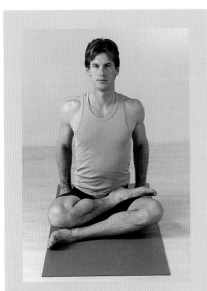

ALTERNATIVE

If you are unable to place your left foot on top of the upper right thigh, then place the left foot in front of the right knee, resting it on the floor. Bring the left arm back to your side. With practice your hips will open, and it is important to be patient.

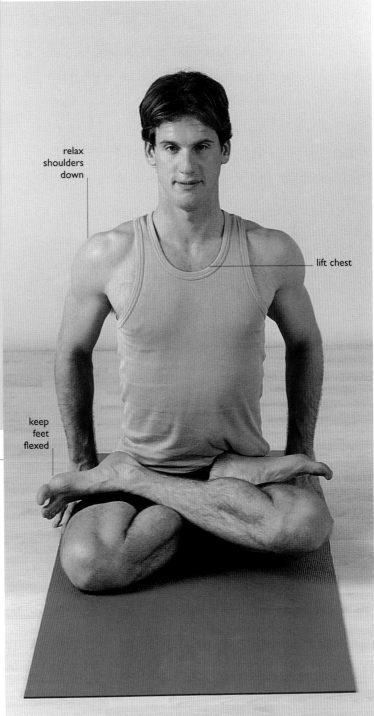

relax shoulders down

lift chest

keep feet flexed

2 Exhaling, grasp your left ankle with your left hand and fold your left leg in toward your belly. Place the left foot on top of the upper right thigh, keeping the left foot flexed. Press the right knee down toward the floor, bringing the sitting bones forward if necessary. Do not force both knees to the floor. Bring your left arm back to your side and gaze forward. Hold *Padmasana 1* for 10 breaths before moving into *Padmasana 2* (*pp.142–143*), if you feel able, or *Savasana* (*p.144*).

PADMASANA 2
Lotus 2

Once you have mastered *Padmasana 1,* you are ready to extend the sequence by incorporating the second variation of the lotus, which is shown here. This particular variant not only releases the hips, but also stretches the spine and exercises the shoulder muscles. Hold the full pose for 10 breaths.

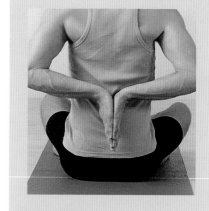

ALTERNATIVE
If you are unable to place your hands in prayer position, press your palms together and point your fingertips down, so your thumbs touch your spine.

pull back the front shoulder

lift chest

Press your palms together and reach up with the fingers. Keep the shoulder blades down.

1 Start from the lotus 1 full pose (*see p.141*). Inhaling, bend your arms behind your back and bring the hands together in prayer form with fingertips pointing upward and your little fingers touching the spine. Press the palms together and gaze straight ahead.

2 Exhaling, fold your body forward, keeping your hands in prayer position behind your back. If possible, touch the floor with your forehead. Draw down the back of the body to move the sitting bones toward the floor. Gaze downward. Hold the full pose for 10 breaths, before releasing and sitting up straight, ready to lie on your back in *Savasana* [*p.144*].

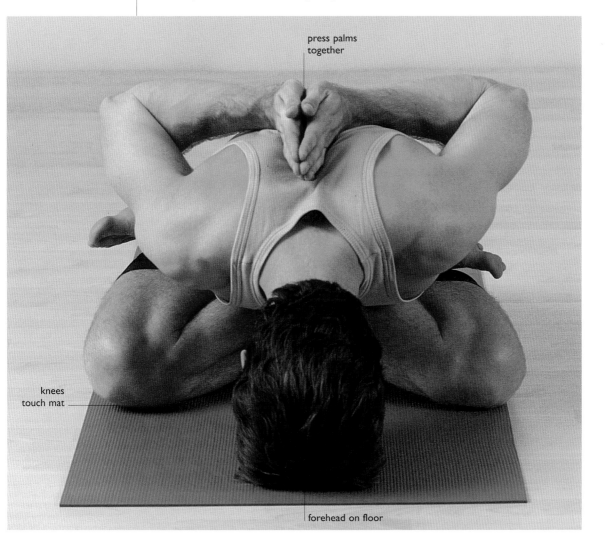

press palms
together

knees
touch mat

forehead on floor

SAVASANA
Corpse

The final pose in every program, *Savasana* allows you to enter a meditative state while resting your body. In Sanskrit *sava* means "corpse," and this pose requires you to relax completely by lying perfectly still, and to focus the mind on internal sensation to achieve a meditative state. When your mind begins to wander, as it will do, note that it is wandering and bring your attention back to the present moment of pure sensation. Remain in this pose for 10 to 15 minutes.

Exhaling, lay down flat on your back with your arms and legs making a 30° angle to the body. Let your hands and feet fall out to the side, palms facing upward. Draw the shoulders down the back. Breathe naturally, close your eyes, and allow the weight of the body to melt into the floor.

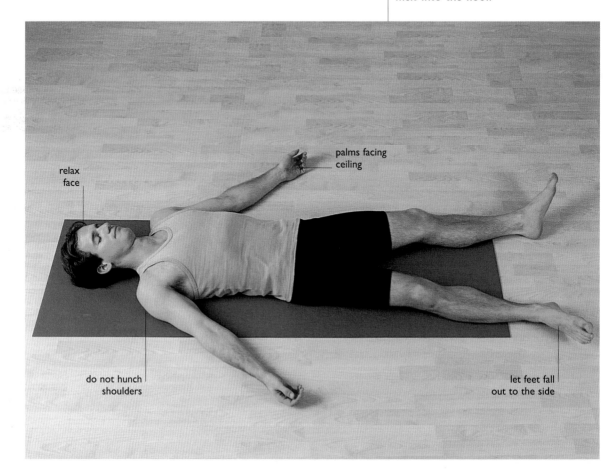

relax face

palms facing ceiling

do not hunch shoulders

let feet fall out to the side

THE PROGRAMS

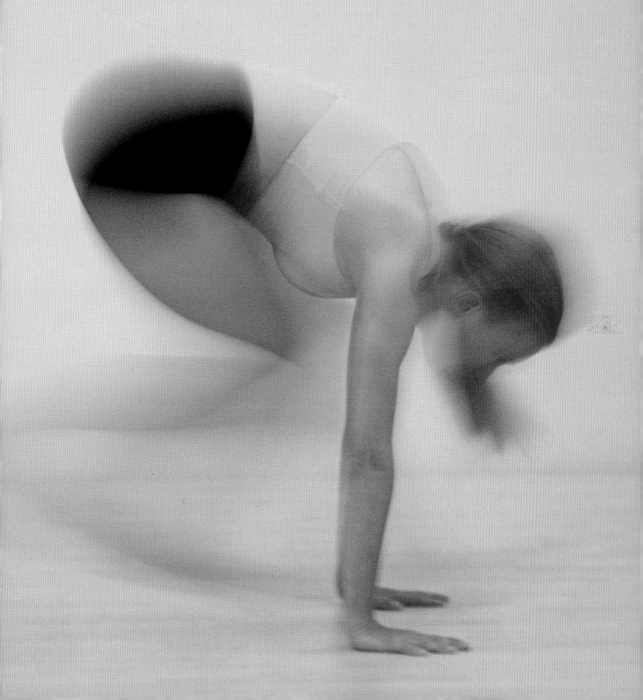

30-MINUTE PROGRAM

The following program is designed to give you a complete yoga practice if you have only half an hour to spare. It is the least strenuous of the three programs detailed. Before beginning, you need to warm up your body. Choose one sitting and one standing warm-up exercise from the four shown on pages 14–17. After this, do the Sun Salutation A sequence twice (*pp.20–29*) and the Sun Salutation B twice (*pp.30–41*). Next, jump out to the side (*pp.46–47*) and begin the program. Practice the right side and then the left side in all bilateral postures, and refer to the main text for all the steps in the postures and transition moves until you know them well.

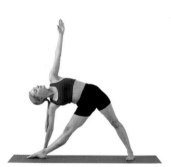

1 Utthita Trikonasana
(*pp.48–49*)

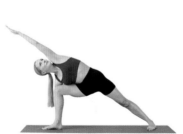

2 Utthita Parsvakonasana
(*pp.52–53*)

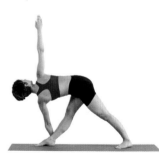

3 Parivrtta Trikonasana
(*pp.62–63*)

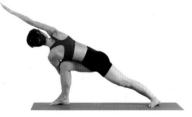

4 Parivrtta Parsvakonasana
(*pp.60–61*)

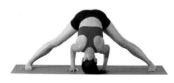

5 Prasarita Padottanasana A
(*pp.64–65*)

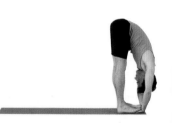

6 Padangusthasana & Padahastasana
(*pp.68–71*)

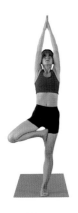

TRANSITION MOVE

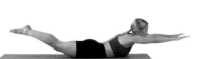

TRANSITION MOVE

7 Vrksasana
(pp.72–73)

8 Standing to Lying on Belly
(pp.82–83)

9 Salabhasana
(pp.84–85)

10 Bow to Sitting
(pp.90–93)

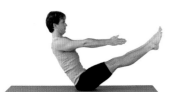

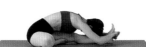

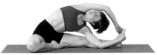

11 Navasana
(pp.104–105)

12 Janu Sirsasana
(pp.114–115)

13 Parivrtta Janu Sirsasana
(pp.116–117)

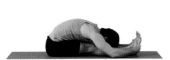

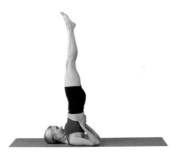

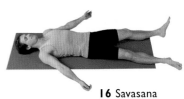

14 Paschimattanasana
(pp.126–127)

15 Salamba Sarvangasana
(pp.136–137)

16 Savasana
(pp.144)

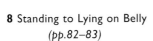

60-MINUTE PROGRAM

This program will give you a complete yoga practice in one hour. Before beginning this 60-minute dynamic yoga program, warm up your body with one sitting and one standing warm-up exercise (*see pp.14–17*). Continue to warm up your body by doing Sun Salutation A three times (*pp.20–29*), and Sun Salutation B (*pp.30–41*) three times. Next, jump out to the side (*pp.46–47*) and begin the program. Practice the right side and then the left side in all bilateral postures, and refer to the main text for any steps in the postures and transition moves of which you are unsure.

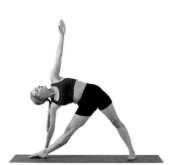

1 Utthita Trikonasana
(*pp.48–49*)

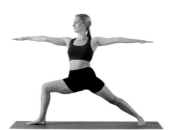

2 Virabhadrasana B
(*pp.50–51*)

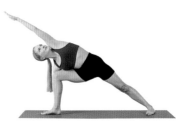

3 Utthita Parsvakonasana
(*pp.52–53*)

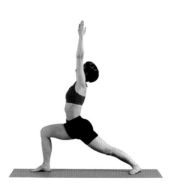

4 Virabhadrasana A
(*pp.58–59*)

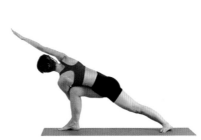

5 Parivrtta Parsvakonasana
(*pp.60–61*)

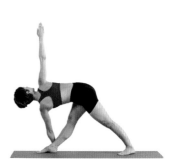

6 Parivrtta Trikonasana
(*pp.62–63*)

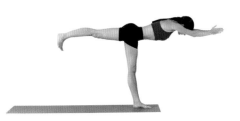

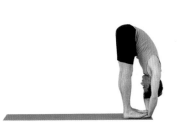

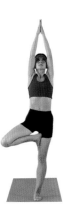

7 Prasarita Padottanasana A
(pp.64–67)

8 Padangusthasana & Padahastasana
(pp.68–71)

9 Vrksasana
(pp.72–73)

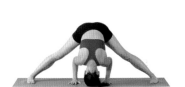

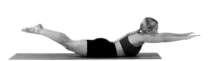

10 Virabhadrasana C
(pp.74–75)

TRANSITION MOVE
11 Standing to Lying on Belly
(pp.82–83)

12 Salabhasana
(pp.84–85)

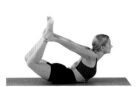

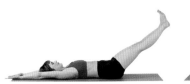

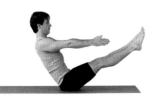

13 Dhanurasana
(pp.88–89)

TRANSITION MOVE
14 Bow to Sitting
(pp.90–91)

15 Urdhva Prasarita Padasana
(pp.96–97)

16 Navasana
(pp.104–105)

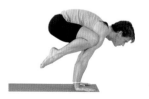

TRANSITION MOVE

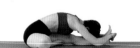

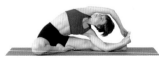

17 Bakasana
(pp.106–107)

18 Crane to Sitting
(pp.108–111)

19 Janu Sirsasana
(pp.114–115)

20 Parivrtta Janu Sirsasana
(pp.116–117)

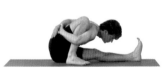

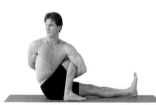

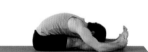

21 Marichyasana A
(pp.122–123)

22 Marichyasana C
(pp.124–125)

23 Paschimattanasana
(pp.126–127)

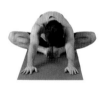

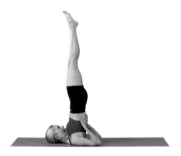

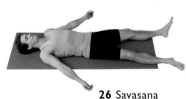

24 Baddha Konasana
(pp.128–129)

25 Salamba Sarvangasana
(pp.136–137)

26 Savasana
(pp.144)

90-MINUTE PROGRAM

The following program is designed to give you a complete yoga practice over 90 minutes. It includes all the *asanas* in the book and is the most strenuous of the three programs. Before beginning this program, warm up your body with both sitting and both standing warm-up exercises (*see pp.14–17*). Continue with five Sun Salutation A sequences (*pp.20–29*), and five Sun Salutation B (*pp.30–41*). Next, jump out to the side (*pp.46–47*) and begin the program. Practice the right side and then the left in all bilateral postures, and refer to the main text for any steps in the postures or transition moves of which you are uncertain.

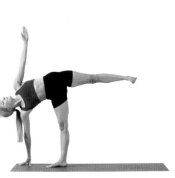

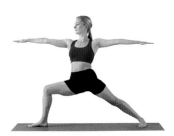

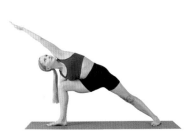

1 Utthita Trikonasana
(*pp.48–49*)

2 Virabhadrasana B
(*pp.50–51*)

3 Utthita Parsvakonasana
(*pp.52–53*)

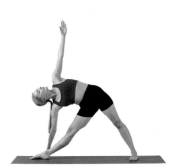

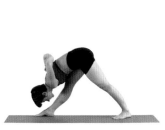

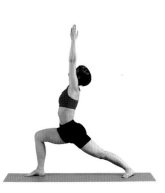

4 Ardha Chandrasana
(*pp.54–55*)

5 Parsvottanasana
(*pp.56–57*)

6 Virabhadrasana A
(*pp.58–59*)

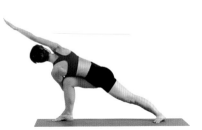

7 Parivrtta Parsvakonasana
(pp.60–61)

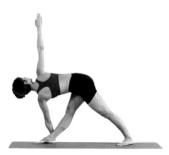

8 Parivrtta Trikonasana
(pp.62–63)

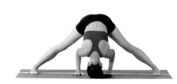

9 Prasarita Padottanasana A
(pp.64–67)

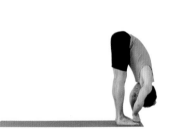

10 Padangusthasana
(pp.68–71)

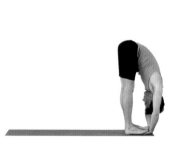

11 Padahastasana
(pp.68–71)

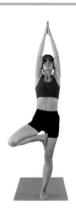

12 Vrksasana
(pp.72–73)

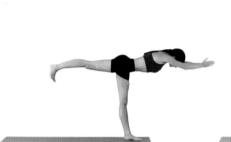

13 Virabhadrasana C
(pp.74–75)

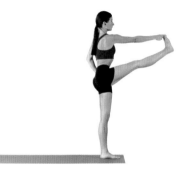

14 Utthita Hasta Padangusthasana
(pp.76–79)

TRANSITION MOVE

15 Standing to Lying on Belly
(pp.82–83)

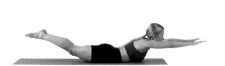

16 Salabhasana
(pp.84–85)

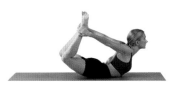

17 Dhanurasana
(pp.88–89)

TRANSITION MOVE

18 Bow to Sitting
(pp.90–93)

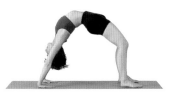

19 Urdhva Dhanurasana
(pp.94–95)

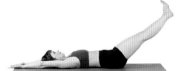

20 Urdhva Prasarita Padasana
(pp.96–97)

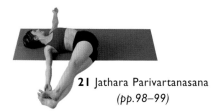

21 Jathara Parivartanasana
(pp.98–99)

TRANSITION MOVE

22 Lying on Back to Sitting
(pp.100–101)

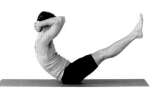

23 Ardha Navasana
(pp.102–103)

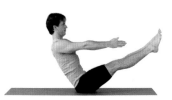

24 Paripurna Navasana
(pp.104–105)

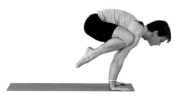

TRANSITION MOVE

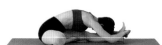

25 Bakasana
(pp.106–107)

26 Crane to Sitting
(pp.108–111)

27 Janu Sirsasana
(pp.114–115)

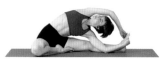

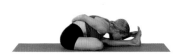

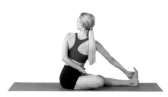

28 Parivrtta Janu Sirsasana
(pp.116–117)

29 Ardha Baddha Padma Paschimattanasana
(pp.118–119)

30 Ardha Matsyendrasana
(pp.120–121)

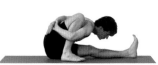

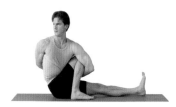

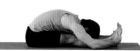

31 Marichyasana A
(pp.122–123)

32 Marichyasana C
(pp.124–125)

33 Paschimattanasana
(pp.126–127)

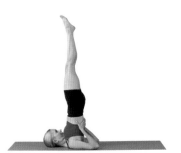
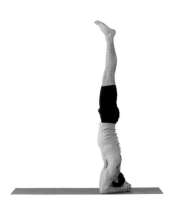
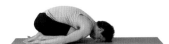

34 Baddha Konasana
(pp.128–129)

35 Salamba Sirsasana
(pp.132–134)

36 Balasana
(pp.135)

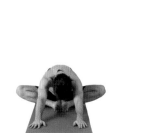
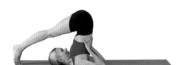
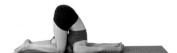

37 Salamba Sarvangasana
(pp.136–137)

38 Halasana
(pp.138–139)

39 Karnapidasana
(pp.138–139)

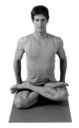

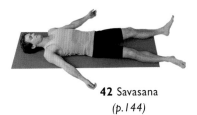

40 Padmasana 1
(pp.140–141)

41 Padmasana 2
(pp.142–143)

42 Savasana
(p.144)

FINDING A YOGA TEACHER

Dynamic is just one wonderful way of describing a style of yoga that uses the Sun Salutations to link several postures, while incorporating the breath and the *bandhas*. So a yoga teacher who adheres to its basic principles may also describe his or her class as: power flow, Ashtanga flow, Hatha flow, or Vinyasa flow. Each of these classes can be unique in its sequence of postures.

A good yoga teacher is someone who combines sensitivity, creativity, and inspiration with technical knowledge and experience. The following online yoga websites offer teacher directories for a wide range of yoga styles: www.yogasite.com; www.yogadirectory.com; www.yogafinder.com. If you would like to contact me directly, look me up online at www.dynamicyoga.net.

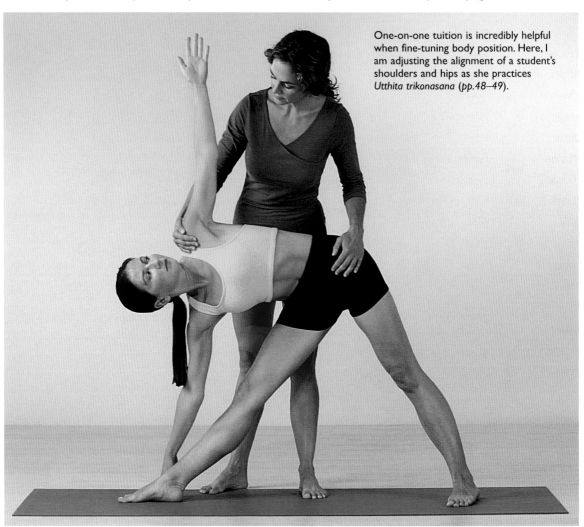

One-on-one tuition is incredibly helpful when fine-tuning body position. Here, I am adjusting the alignment of a student's shoulders and hips as she practices *Utthita trikonasana* (pp.48–49).

GLOSSARY OF SANSKRIT TERMS

adho mukha	face downward	*parivrtta*	revolved
ahimsa	non-violence	*parsva*	side
angustha	big toe	*paschimattana*	posterior stretch
aparigraha	non-attachment	*prana*	breath
ardha	half	*pranayama*	rhythmic control of breath
asana	posture	*prasarita*	expanded
ashtanga	eight limbs	*pratyahara*	merging of the senses
asteya	non-stealing	*purva*	east
brahmacharya	purity	*purvottana*	anterior stretch
baddha	bound	*raja–yoga*	path of meditation
baka	crane	*salabha*	locust
bandha	lock	*santosha*	contentment
bhakti	worship	*satya*	truth
chandra	moon	*sarvanga*	whole body
chaturanga	number four	*saucha*	purity
dhanu	bow	*sava*	corpse
dharana	concentration	*setu*	bridge
dhyana	meditation	*sirsa*	head
dhanda	staff	*surya*	sun
hala	plow	*svadhaya*	self-study
hasta	hand	*svana*	dog
hatha	force	*tada*	mountain
jathara	abdomen	*tapas*	austerity
janu	knee	*trikona*	triangle
karma	action	*uddiyana*	flying upward
karna–pida	pressure around the ear	*ujjayi*	victorious
kona	angle	*urdhva mukha*	face upward
mula	root	*utkata*	fierce
niyama	self-purification	*uttana*	intense stretch
namaskara	honorable salutation	*utthita*	extended
nava	boat	*virabhadra*	warrior
pada	foot	*vrksa*	tree
padangustha	big toe	*yama*	ethical disciplines
padma	lotus	*yoga*	union

INDEX

ACKNOWLEDGMENTS

Author acknowledgements

I want to thank the great love in my life, Kevin Welch, for his encouragement and faith; my soulmate, Kristi Hagen, for everything that words cannot describe; my parents, Jocelyn and Stewart, for allowing my curious spirit to flourish; my sister, Julie Lutz, for her endless support in everything I have done; and my favorite brother, David, for giving me a sense of humor.

I also want to thank all of the models: Emma, Sophie, Imogen, and especially Jamie Lindsay for also helping create the context of the book. I want to thank the editor, Jane Laing, for all her creative talent and the rest of the DK team: Karen Sawyer, Jenny Jones, Miranda Harvey, Gillian Roberts, and Mary-Clare Jerram for their tremendous help and belief in me. Also, a big thanks to the photographer, Russell Sadur, for his expertise and humor, and to my dear friend, Andy Larson, for all of his help. Finally, I thank all of the yoga teachers that have helped me along my path.

Publisher's acknowledgments

The publisher would like to thank Helen Ridge for help with the editing, Maggie McCormick for proof-reading, Anna Grapes for picture research, and Dorothy Frame for the index.

Picture credits

The publisher would like to thank the following for their kind permission to reproduce their photographs:
9: Charles Walker Collection; 8: from *Children Just Like Me – Celebration!* by Barnabas and Anabel Kindersley, published by Dorling Kindersley
All other images © Dorling Kindersley
For further information see: www.dkimages.com

Commissioned photography

Photographer: Russell Sadur
Photographer's assistant: Nina Duncan

Models: Kia Meaux, Emma Catto, Imogen Ashby, Sophie Anns, and Jamie Lindsay
Set builder: Mike Cooper
Hair and makeup: Chloe Butcher

All the women's sports and leisure clothing used in the photoshoot was provided by Carita House. It is from their DANS*EZ SUPPLEX RANGE.
For a free mail order catalogue, please contact:
Carita House
Stapeley
Nantwich
Cheshire CW5 7LJ
tel: 01270 627722
fax: 01270 626684
email: action@caritahouse.com
www.caritahouse.com

All the exercise mats used in the photoshoot were supplied by Hugger Mugger Yoga Products. They are Standard Tapas mat, which provide a stable, non-slip surface for yoga practice.
You can obtain these mats from:
Hugger Mugger Yoga Products
3937 So 500 W
Salt Lake City
Utah 84123
tel: 800 473 4888
fax: 801 268 2629
www.huggermugger.com
and also from:
Hugger Mugger Yoga Products
12 Roseneath Place
Edinburgh
EH9 1JB
tel/fax: 0131 221 9977
email: yme@ednet.co.uk
www.yoga.co.uk